NEUROLOGY - LABORATORY AND CLINICAL
RESEARCH DEVELOPMENTS

NEUROPLASTICITY IN THE AUDITORY BRAINSTEM: FROM PHYSIOLOGY TO THE DRUG THERAPY

NEUROLOGY – LABORATORY AND CLINICAL RESEARCH DEVELOPMENTS

Additional books in this series can be found on Nova's website
under the Series tab.

Additional E-books in this series can be found on Nova's website
under the E-book tab.

PHARMACOLOGY - RESEARCH, SAFETY TESTING AND REGULATION

Additional books in this series can be found on Nova's website
under the Series tab.

Additional E-books in this series can be found on Nova's website
under the E-book tab.

NEUROLOGY - LABORATORY AND CLINICAL
RESEARCH DEVELOPMENTS

NEUROPLASTICITY IN THE AUDITORY BRAINSTEM: FROM PHYSIOLOGY TO THE DRUG THERAPY

ANGELO SALAMI
EDITOR

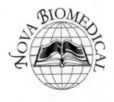

Nova Science Publishers, Inc.
New York

MW

For permission to use material from this book please contact us:
Telephone 631-231-7269; Fax 631-231-8175
Web Site: http://www.novapublishers.com

NOTICE TO THE READER

The Publisher has taken reasonable care in the preparation of this book, but makes no expressed or implied warranty of any kind and assumes no responsibility for any errors or omissions. No liability is assumed for incidental or consequential damages in connection with or arising out of information contained in this book. The Publisher shall not be liable for any special, consequential, or exemplary damages resulting, in whole or in part, from the readers' use of, or reliance upon, this material. Any parts of this book based on government reports are so indicated and copyright is claimed for those parts to the extent applicable to compilations of such works.

Independent verification should be sought for any data, advice or recommendations contained in this book. In addition, no responsibility is assumed by the publisher for any injury and/or damage to persons or property arising from any methods, products, instructions, ideas or otherwise contained in this publication.

This publication is designed to provide accurate and authoritative information with regard to the subject matter covered herein. It is sold with the clear understanding that the Publisher is not engaged in rendering legal or any other professional services. If legal or any other expert assistance is required, the services of a competent person should be sought. FROM A DECLARATION OF PARTICIPANTS JOINTLY ADOPTED BY A COMMITTEE OF THE AMERICAN BAR ASSOCIATION AND A COMMITTEE OF PUBLISHERS.

Additional color graphics may be available in the e-book version of this book.

Library of Congress Cataloging-in-Publication Data

Neuroplasticity in the auditory brainstem from physiology to the drug therapy / editor, Angelo Salami.
       p. ; cm.
   Includes bibliographical references and index.
   ISBN 978-1-61761-949-6 (hardcover)
   1. Auditory pathways. 2. Neuroplasticity. 3. Brain stem. 4. Cochlear implants. I. Salami, Angelo.
   [DNLM: 1. Auditory Pathways--physiology. 2. Brain Stem--physiology. 3. Neuronal Plasticity--drug effects. 4. Neuronal Plasticity--physiology. WV 272]
   QP461.N48 2010
   612.8'5--dc22
                                                                                      2010036145

Published by Nova Science Publishers, Inc. † *New York*

3/12/12

Contents

Contents

Introduction

Today, in contrast with past knowledge, it is known that the brain is actually capable of changing and developing throughout a lifetime. Recent expereices highlight as the human brain is incredibly adaptive. Our mental capacity is astonishingly large, and our ability to process widely varied information and complex new experiences with relative ease can often be surprising. The brain's ability to act and react in ever-changing ways is known as neuroplasticity. Neuroplasticity (also referred to as brain plasticity, cortical plasticity or cortical re-mapping) is the changing of neurons, the organization of their networks, and their function via new experiences.

Decades of research have now shown that these changes can profoundly alter the pattern of neuronal activation in response to experience. According to the theory of neuroplasticity, thinking, learning, acting and hearing can change both the brain's physical structure and functional organization according to the peripheral stimuli.

One of the fundamental principles of how neuroplasticity functions is linked to the concept of synaptic pruning, the idea that individual connections within the brain are constantly being removed or recreated, largely dependent upon how they are used.

One of the ways neuroplasticity may work is when people have traumatic brain injuries. Even part of the brain could be damaged or removed and this doesn't necessarily mean the function that that part tends to govern is lost forever. It can mean that, but the brain may adapt by growing new synapses to restore a certain type of function. Such knowledge has made it extremely clear that things like physical and occupational therapy are vital during early recovery from stroke. Encouraging the brain to exhibit neuroplasticity is very important in achieving best recovery results.

The aim of this book was to report the last knowledge on the neuroplasticity in the auditory brainstem: from physiology to the drug therapy.

I'm pleased and honored for the high value of the authors which have contributed to this book. In particular in the first chapter prof. O. Michel have described the anatomy of the central auditory pathway, in the second chapter the physiology has been accurately reported by prof. A. Ryan, in the third chapter the ENT Clinic of Genoa have highlighted the neurobiology, Prof. P. Gil-Loyzaga have shown the plastic change in the auditory system after hearing loss while Prof. M. Casselbrant have described the correlation between hearing loss and balance dysfunction in children, in chapter 6 Prof. H.O. Seung have presented the effect of brain plasticity on the results of cochlear implantation, while the last three chapters have regarded the description of new approaches in the treatment of hearing loss (Dr Manini, Prof. A. Salami and Prof. R. Salvi).

Angelo Salami

In: Neuroplasticity in the Auditory Brainstem   ISBN 978-1-61761-949-6
Editor: Angelo Salami, pp. 1-12   © 2011 Nova Science Publishers, Inc.

Chapter I

Anatomy of the Auditory Pathway

Olaf Michel[*]

Universitair Ziekenhuis, Brussel, Belgium

Abstract

The human auditory system has inputs from both ears, which are connected by cross-over fibers from both ascending pathways. Both pathways from each ear have parallel organized processing but still with connection to the other site. Within both pathways distinct groups of neurons - nuclei - are embedded. These nuclei also have neuronal interconnections, allowing feed-back loops in the ascending as well as in the descending pathway.

The uppermost fundamental property of the auditory nervous system is its tonotopic organization from the cochlea to the auditory cortex, which can continuously be recognized by anatomical findings and by physiological experiments.

The auditory pathway includes 4 neurons from the hair cell to the auditory cortex. The spiral ganglion cell axons from the cochlea terminate in the cochlear nuclei, from which they project in one major pathway to the

---

[*] Correspondance: Prof. Dr. O. Michel, Universitair Ziekenhuis - Vrije Universiteit Brussel UZ-VUB, Laarbeeklaan 101, B-1090 Brüssel, Tel.: +32-2-477 6889/6888, Fax: +32-2-477 6880, Email: OMichel@uzbrussel.de

superior olive (SO) and in another pathway from the ventral cochlear nucleus (VCN) to the medial nucleus of the trapezoid body (TB) and the lateral superior olive. The trapezoid body forms the most important transverse auditory tract.

From the superior olive fibers project via the lateral lemniscus to the nucleus of the lateral lemniscus and the inferior colliculus, where all of the brainstem auditory pathways converge. From here projections can be found to the thalamus (particularly the medial geniculate nucleus), from where they are relayed to the auditory cortex.

Up to the auditory cortex the tonotopic (or cochleotopic) pattern can be followed in the cytoarchitecture. Nevertheless, the input from two ears and the cross-linked pathways allow the detection of differences in sound intensity and thus the localization of sound sources.

1. The Inner Ear

The inner hair cells (IHC) are the primary sensory cells transforming physical energy into electrical impulses. They are innervated by afferent fibres which are primarily unmyelinated. After leaving the neural endings the afferent fibers pass the habenula perforata, a series of tiny holes beneath the inner hair cells towards the bony modiolus. From this point on, they got a myelin sheath. After a short course in the modiolus, the peripheral process joins is cell body (perikaryon) in the spiral ganglion (SG). There are about 23,000 of fibers in man, and the greater number of them - about 95 percent - innervate the inner hair cells. The remainder cross the tunnel of Corti to innervate the outer hair cells (OHC). On their way they pick up collaterals from many of the hair cell they go by. The innervation of the OHC is much more diffuse and overlapping than is the case for IHC, which are sharply tuned to their fibers.

The neurons of the SG are called bipolar cells because they have two branches of fibres that extend from opposite ends of the cell body. Only the shorter, peripheral fibers extend to the bases of the inner and outer hair cells.

The longer central axons (also called the primary auditory fibers) form at least the acoustic (cochlear) nerve (AN). The perikarya, which are located in the SG the modiolus of the cochlea, are therefore the first neurons of the ascendant auditory pathway, which includes at least four neurons.

2. The Auditory Nerve

The auditory nerve (AN, also called cochlear nerve, acoustic nerve) is consequently formed by the longer central processes of the bipolar cochlear neurons, which originate from the spiral ganglion (SG). The fibers of the AN twist like the cords of a rope within the modiolar section of the cochlea and are myelinated throughout their length. The fibers of the AN become part of the vestibulocochlear-nerve (VIIIth cranial nerve), which passes the inner auditory canal (IAC). Just before entering the cranial cavity Schwann cells are replaced by neuroglia cells. The AN transverses together with the facial nerve the cerebellopontine angle (CPA) to the medulla.

In the internal auditory meatus the AN is situated inferior to the facial nerve within the anterior-inferior quadrant and immediately anterior to the inferior vestibular nerve. Between cochlea and the medulla the AN has in man a length about 5 mm. The size of the acoustic nerve varies in different species in length and in axon counts.

3. The Central Auditory Pathway

3.1. The Cochlear Nuclear Complex (CNC)

The AN enters the upper medulla immediately superficial to the inferior cerebellar peduncle (vestibulocochlear nerve root entry zone or pontomedullary junction).

Each afferent acoustic fiber from the AN bifurcates immediately upon entering and sends a branch to each of the two primary cochlear nuclei (CN, nucleus cochlearis).

These nuclei are groups of nerve cell bodies similar to a peripheral ganglion [Moore, 2000]. Nuclei of such type are found moreover in different places in the auditory pathway (AP) and the central nervous system (CNS) in general. For magnet resonance imaging (MRI) purposes, these nuclei in the upper medulla have been referred to as the cochlear nuclear complex (CNC), which images is tubular structure, 8 mm in length and about 3 mm thick [Gebarski et al., 1993].

The ventral branch of the fibers of the AN divides again to penetrate the anterior (AVCN) and posterior (PVCN) divisions of the ventral cochlear nucleus (VCN), whereas the dorsal branch penetrates the dorsal cochlear nucleus (DCN) without dividing. Nearly all auditory nerve fibers terminate within the CNC.

Within all of these three primary nuclei there is an orderly arrangement of cellular endings which corresponds directly with the locus within the cochlear spiral of the hair cells that they innervate. The result is a strict tonotopic arrangement. The basal end of the cochlea, which encodes high frequencies, projects the most dorsally and the apical end of the cochlea, which encodes low frequencies, most ventrally to the VCN. The fibers of the lower basal end of the cochlear show some deviation from this orderly pattern with a more diffuse distribution within the nuclei.

This tonotopic or "cochleotopic" arrangement of fibers is maintained throughout the auditory pathway. Thus, tonotopic projection is of utmost importance for understanding the specific organization of the auditory pathway and the principles which underlay various pathophysiological conditions [Hackney, 1987].

Within the AVCN, PVCN and DCN specializations are found neuroanatomically, which correspond to different cell structures and functional properties. The division in different regions is based on the distribution of the predominant cell types and follows therefore the cytoarchitectonic structure [Dublin, 1982].

In the AVCN, stellate neurons and bushy cells prevail. The AN fibers terminate on the cell bodies of the bushy cells with large calyceal endings, which are named end bulbs of Held. The endings engulf a large portion of the postsynaptic cellular surface of the bushy cells. The end bulbs appear specialized for rapid transmission of nerve impulses from the cochlea. Small bouton endings were also found, but their significance is largely unknown.

The bushy cells have a restricted distribution in the AVCN. Spherical bushy cells (SBC) and globular bushy cells (GBC), which are found in the more caudal region of the AVCN in and around the nerve root area, have been identified. A SBC and a GBC pathway can be distinguished, which provide direct excitatory and indirect inhibitory input, respectively, to binaural nuclei in the SOC. SBCs are the most numerous projection neurons of the CN .

In the caudal pole of the PVCN, one of the major cell groups is the so called octopus cell. Their dendritic branches extend across the afferents converging to enter the DCN. Octopus cells were found to be innervated from collaterals of the descending branch of the cochlear nerve as well. The collaterals terminate as bouton type endings on the dendrites and on the bodies of the cells; each cell and its dendrites are innervated by collaterals arising from many descending branch axons.

Within the CNC the first auditory synapses occur. From these 3 medulla nuclei on, the so called binaural brain stem pathway initiates and extends finally to the cerebral cortex. Nevertheless, each cochlear nucleus (CN) receives fibers only from the ear of the same side.

The initial divergence of the fibers from the AN into three branches to the AVCN, PVCN and DCN continues in three main routes of the ascending pathway. These three major bundles are the ventral acoustic stria, the dorsal acoustic stria and the intermediate acoustic stria (stria of Held).

The ventral acoustic stria or trapezoid body (TB) is a major transverse auditory tract constituting a broad fiber plate in the ventral pons. The neuron axons cross from the AVCN in the TB to the contralateral side. The bushy cells of the AVCN project directly on the ipsilateral and contralateral medial superior olivary nucleus (MSO), which is situated in the medulla oblongata (MO). Also cells from the PVCN reach by this pathway major cell groups of the superior olivary complex (SOC).

The dorsal acoustic stria (stria of Monakow) is a pathway, which runs from the DCN to the contralateral central nucleus of the inferior colliculus (IC) but projects to the nuclei of the lateral lemniscus (LL) as well.

The intermediate acoustic stria (stria of Held) originates mainly from the PCVN and projects to periolivary cell groups bilaterally.

The DCN also receives a variety of inputs form other auditory nuclei as well as nonauditory centers. For example, the DCN receives descending input from the inferior colliculus (IC) bilaterally, from the ventral cochlear nucleus (VCN), from the cerebellum, from the reticular formation, and probably from several other midbrain and brainstem regions. Cells in the dorsal cochlear nucleus have complex coding characteristics.

These neuroanatomical relations are supposed to have functional importance in the formation of tinnitus other than cochlear origin, the so called somatogenic tinnitus [Levine, 1999]. 4 different cranial nerves (V, VII, IX, and X) converge to the region of the common spinal tract (CST) namely the ipsilateral dorsolateral lower medulla and upper cervical spinal cord. This region has been referred to as the "medullary somatosensory nuclei" (MSN). This region of anatomical convergence - MSN - is directly connected by fibers with the DSN as shown in cats and rats. However, there are yet no studies, which would confirm also in humans a pathway from the cuneate/spinal tract of V to the ipsilateral DCN. Additionally, the cytoarchitecture of the human DCN differs from that of many other mammals. The IC as another possible site in the auditory pathway is regarded to be a less likely location for a somatic-auditory interaction for not otogenic tinnitus.

From the PVCN fibers cross obliquely as the posterior acoustic striae. Collaterals of these fibers (or other axons) transverse the midline in the intermediate acoustic stria (of Held) and issue collaterals to the periolivary nuclei. Most fibers ascend as the lateral lemniscus (LL) to the IC at the midbrain. There, these second neurons make synapse with the third neuron. Some fibers from the DCN, which pass in the ipsilateral LL, also go directly to the medial geniculate nucleus (MGN) [Shinohara et al., 2004].

3.2. Superior Olivary Complex (SOC)

The superior olivary complex (SOC) consists of a number of more or less distinct cell groups, which form three major nuclei. A lateral (LSO) and a medial superior olivary (MSO) nucleus and a medial nucleus of the trapezoid body (MNTB) can be distinguished. The LSO and MSO are surrounded by the smaller cell groups of the pre- and periolivary nuclei.

The MSO is the largest of the nuclei in the auditory pathway and contains approximately 15,500 neurons in humans. It is a dorsoventrally aligned sheet of cells with bipolar dendrites. The medially radiating dendrites receive input from the contralateral AVCN and the lateral dendrites are innervated by fibers from the ipsilateral AVCN. Thus in the MSO, binaural information first converges, making a first comparison between the responses of both the two ears possible. The axonal arbors of the VCN inputs to the MSO are tonotopically constrained. Mostly low frequencies are represented in the MSO. The primary output of MSO is into the ipsilateral lemniscus lateralis (LL).

The MSO receives fibers not only from both of the cochlear nuclei (CN) but also from the nucleus of the TB.

The MNTB, which is situated medial to the MSO, receives fibers from the bushy cells of the contralateral VCN. They form large end-bulbs on the cells. The AVCN projects not only fibers to the medial nucleus of the trapezoid body (MNTB) but to the LSO as well.

The LSO receives an ipsilateral excitatory input from cells in the VCN which respond best to high frequencies. The contralateral input to these cells is disynaptic. The LSO receives input from both cochlear nuclei - from ipsilateral AVCN spherical bushy cells and contralateral AVCN globular bushy cells via the ipsilateral MNTB. Thus, the neurons of the LSO get excitatory input from the ipsilateral ear and inhibitory input from the contralateral ear.

The major outflow from the LSO neurons is into the LL bilaterally, to terminate in the inferior colliculus (IC). Some of these fibers reach the medial geniculate body (MGN) without synapsing in the inferior colliculus (IC). Some fibers from the DCN and some of the fibers from the PVCN bypass the SOC and go also directly to the MGN.

In the region of the superior olivary nuclei there are between 6 and 9 smaller dispersed cell groups which form the periolivary nuclei and which also receive bilateral input from the cochlear nuclei (CN) and both the ascending and descending auditory pathways. These nuclei form the source of the olivocochlear bundle (OCB), which innervates the cochlea in the descending AP.

Additional projection targets include the dorsal and ventral nuclei of the LL (DNLL and VNLL). DNLL and VNLL are embedded within the LL. They represent a synaptic station where a part of the fibers were redirected towards the contralateral LL or receive fibers from the contralateral DCN. The DNLL receives afferents from cells located within the SOC as well as the DNLL. The VCLL receives afferents from the contralateral VCN and a few from the SOC [Harrison, 1987; Reuss, 2000].

3.3. Inferior Colliculus (IC)

Projections from all of the nuclei mentioned above converge on the inferior colliculus (IC), predominantly fibers within the lateral lemniscus (LL) and still in a tonotopic pattern. In addition, direct projections from the contralateral AVCN converge on the same region of the IC that receives olivary (SOC) input. Most of the cells receive in addition descending input from the midbrain and other regions of the central nervous system (CNS) e.g. somatosensory and vocalization systems as well as the cerebellum. Therefore, the IC is an essential auditory relay and auditory reflex centre in the auditory pathway [Aitkin et al., 1993].

The IC itself can be divided in three parts: the central nucleus of IC (ICC), the dorsal (ICD) and lateral cortex (ICL) or ICX with the inclusion of external nuclei in the area rostral and venteromedial to the the ICC. Each nucleus has unique afferent and efferent connections.

The ICC is the principal way station for ascending auditory information in the IC. It has been identified as the relay nucleus for auditory information transmitted via the LL from all brainstem nuclei, predominantly projections from the DCN and the VCN, from the SOC and the nuclei from the LL. The ICC is reciprocally connected with the contralateral ICC and projects as well to the ipsilateral ICX [Huffman et al., 1990]. Ascending projections are primarily to the ventral division of the medial geniculate body (MGN).

The predominant neuron in the ICC is a disc shaped cell with dendritic trees orientated in alignments with the incoming afferent fibers and parallel to one another in a laminar organization [Hackney, 1987]. A well-defined "cochleotopic" organization within the ICC has been described with iso-frequency contours, which are orientated in parallel planes corresponding to the laminar organization of the fibrodendritic sheets.

The ICD does not receive a major input from other auditors centers but has interacting fibers with other subdivisions within the IC. It has an ascending projection to the medial geniculate nucleus (MGN) and a descending input from the auditory cortex (AC). The ICD has a cortical cytoarchitecture with four layers.

The ICX differs from the other parts of the IC, because it receives in addition a somatosensory input from the dorsal column nuclei, spinal cord and sensory terminal nuclei as well as descending projections from auditory and somatosensory sortices and from the superior colliculus (SC). The cytoarchitecture is similar to the ICD; although in the ICX the largest cells of the IC are found.

The ICX projects fibers to the thalamic area to the medial division of the MGB and to descending acusticomotor systems [Huffman et al., 1990]. In line with to the cytoarchitecture the cells have either auditory or somatosensory response properties or even both.

4. Central Pathways and Cortical Projections

From the IC, both streams of information proceed to the sensory thalamus. The thalamus forms part of the diencephalon which is part of the central nervous system (CNS).

The auditory nucleus of thalamus is the medial geniculate nucleus (MGN) and the lateral division of the posterior group of the thalamic nuclei, also called the medial geniculate complex (MGC) or medial genicular body (MGB). The MGC receives its input from the ipsilateral ICC via the LL. The MGC contains two main cell types –principal cells and Golgi Type 2 cells, which are local interneurons and presumably inhibitory.

In the MGC, ventral (VMGN), dorsal (DMGN) and medial nuclei (MMGN) can be distinguished.

The VMGN is the major thalamic component for the auditory ascending pathway, which is tonotopically organized. His cytoarchitecture consists mainly in principal cells. These principal cells show a laminar fibrodendritic organization along with the parallel orientation of afferent fibers reminiscent of the ICC. The

VMGN receives input from the ICC and sends dense, reciprocal projections to the to the primary auditory cortex (PAC, AI).

The DMGN has a less structured cellular organization as the VMGN. It receives fibres from the ICD and has reciprocal connections to the secondary auditory cortex (AII).

The MMGN consists of medium and small type cells with different dendritic organizations and has therefore a more heterogenic cytoarchitecture compared to the VMGN. The special feature of the MMGN consists in his integration of multisensory input in addition to auditory input. It also receives fibers from the ICX, which is also multisensory. The MMGN makes connections to all the AC areas.

5. The Primary Auditory Cortex (PAC, AI)

The primary auditory cortex (PAC, AI) is located on the banks of the temporal lobes. In man, the PAC is situated on the inner surface of the superior temporal gyrus (of Heschl), placed deep in the Sylvian fissure (Brodmann's area 41) and it is characterized by a high density of granule cells.

The tonotopic organization is maintained all the way to the PAC and also within. Inside Brodmann's area 41 high frequencies are represented posterodorsally and low frequencies are represented anteroventrally. The PAC receives information from both of the cochleae.

Surrounding the "primary" auditory cortex (AI) are a series of "secondary" auditory fields (AII) (e.g. Brodmann's area 22), which may receive direct projections from the MGN, but also connect reciprocally with the PAC as well as with the thalamic nuclei.

The different auditory fields can be distinguished from one another by their structural and functional properties. In humans, "association areas" such as Wernicke's area are of particular importance. Bordering AI and AII is another auditory area (Ep), which is also organized tonotopically. Auditory responses are also found in other zones (e.g. Area of Tunturi, AIII).

In summary, the PAC is one of the most important anatomic portions to the auditory processing, receiving most information from the MGC. Once in AI there is the conclusion of the whole process of coding and decoding of the heard information from both ears.

6. Efferent Projections

Efferent fibers project from the brain to the cochlea in a complex system of pathways, because for each projection of the ascending pathway there is a parallel ascending projection. Thus, the efferent fibers complement those of the ascending auditory pathway. They play a crucial role in the perception of sound constituting an efferent system, or feedback loop, by which nerve impulses, thought to be inhibitory, reach the hair cells.

The descending auditory pathway comprises three major projections from

1. the auditory cortex (AC) to both the MGB and IC,
2. the IC to both cochlear nuclei (CN) and the SOC,
3. the SOC to the cochlea.

6.1. From the AC to both the MBG and IC

The auditory cortex comprises several areas, projecting in different terminal endings within the IC. The majority of these corticocollicular fibers terminate in the ICD and ICX, strictly tonotopically organized as the ascending pathway. The ICC does not receive projections from the AC in many species.

From the AC also projections to the MGN can be found, which are parallel to those to the IC. They are predominantly from pyramidal cells of the AC .

To the MMGN, corticogeniculate fibers can be found from all areas of the AC. A major portion of fibers from the AI terminate in the VMGN, whereas projections from AII terminate in the VMGN and in the DMGN. There are also fibers found, which project from the ectosylvian area (EP) to the DMGN.

Cytoarchitectural studies in several species have shown parallel connections among discrete parts of the AC, IC and MGC, which may form a system of multiple, segregated feed-back-loops. This becomes evident in the connections from each of the other two major descending pathways.

6.2. From the IC to both Cochlear Nuclei (CN) and the SOC

Anatomical studies have shown in correspondence to physiological studies that the IC connections with the SOC play a role in the activity of the olivocochlear bundle (OCB) and thus tuning and response properties of the OHC within the cochlea.

Descending fibers from the IC terminate in the CN bilaterally. The major pathway is from the ICC and to a lesser extend from the ICX and the ICD to the contralateral DCN.

Thus, the CN receive altogether efferent fibers from:

1. SOC (the source of the majority of efferent fibres) arising in the pre- and periolivary nuclei (PON).
2. LL (dorsal and ventral nuclei)
3. Reticular formation (extends into the pons from the medulla)

From the IC also fibers project to parts of the SOC , where they terminate. Some of these fibers target the MNTB, but the target areas slightly differ from species to species.

6.3. From the SOC to the Hair Cells

In the SOC two different cell types based on origin and target locations can be anatomically differentiated, small cells and large cells.

Small cells are found to be located around or within the LSO. They are unmyelinated and project predominantly uncrossed to the ipsilateral inner hair cells (IHC). They synapse predominantly on afferent fiber terminals associated with IHC's. Some fibers have their point of origin around the afferent nuclei of the MSO and MNTB as well as in the pre-olivary and periolivary nuclei.

The others are larger multipolar neurons cells, located around the MSO, which project myelinated fibers to the contralateral outer hair cells (OHC), where they synapse on the cell bodies.

The descending tract formed by these efferent fibers is called the olivocochlear bundle (OCB) and is of special interest to study cochlear micromechanics.. The OCB pass dorsomedially as the peduncle of the SOC. The largest part of the fibers cross the median plane and leave the brain stem with the vestibular nerve joining the AN.

In the cochlea, they cross the inner tunnel of the spiral organ as tunnel fibers and end primarily on the OHC.

In summary, the descending pathway between the auditory cortex and the cochlea is trisynaptic. The reciprocal ascending and descending connections for any pair of nuclei among the IC, SOC and the CN allows a system of multiple feedback loops. Additionally, bilateral projections of the efferent pathway provide links between both ears, whereas short links between the ascending and descending pathway allow loop-in-loop-feedback on a subcortical level in the modification and control of the auditory information.

References

Aitkin, L, Park, V. Audition and the auditory pathway of a vocal New World primate, the common marmoset. *Prog Neurobiol* (1993);41:345-367.

Dublin, WB. The cochlear nuclei revisited. *Otolaryngol Head Neck Surg* (1982);90:744-760.

Gebarski, SS, Tucci, DL, Telian, SA. The cochlear nuclear complex: MR location and abnormalities. *AJNR Am J Neuroradiol* (1993);14:1311-1318.

Hackney, CM. Anatomical features of the auditory pathway from cochlea to cortex. *Br Med Bull* (1987);43:780-801.

Harrison, RV. Auditory science tutorial. III: The role of the ascending pathways. *J Otolaryngol* (1987);16:80-88.

Huffman, RF, Henson, OW, Jr. The descending auditory pathway and acousticomotor systems: connections with the inferior colliculus. *Brain Res Brain Res Rev* (1990);15:295-323.

Levine, RA. Somatic (craniocervical) tinnitus and the dorsal cochlear nucleus hypothesis. *Am J Otolaryngol* (1999);20:351-362.

Moore, JK. Organization of the human superior olivary complex. *Microsc Res Tech* (2000);51:403-412.

Reuss, S. Introduction to the superior olivary complex. *Microsc Res Tech* (2000);51:303-306.

Shinohara, H, Yasutaka, S, Taniguchi, Y, Kominami, R, Kawamata, S. Fiber dissection technique for demonstrating the lateral lemniscus of the human brain. *Okajimas Folia Anat Jpn* (2004);80:115-118.

In: Neuroplasticity in the Auditory Brainstem   ISBN 978-1-61761-949-6
Editor: Angelo Salami, pp. 13-29   © 2011 Nova Science Publishers, Inc.

Chapter II

Phsyiology of the Central Auditory System

Sara Euteneuer[1,4] and Allen F. Ryan[1,2,3,*]
[1]Departments of Surgery/Otolaryngology and
[2]Neuroscience UCSD and [3]VA Medical Center, La Jolla, CA, USA
[4]Department of Otolaryngology, University of Lubeck, Lubeck, Germany

Introduction

Acoustic signals are transduced by the cochlea and encoded by the neurons of the cochlear ganglion. The resulting neural activity is transmitted centrally by the fibers of the auditory nerve. The processing of VIIIth nerve discharge into the perception of hearing is accomplished by the central auditory system, which consists of a series of nuclei in the brainstem and midbrain, and culminates in auditory cortex. From here auditory information is further processed in various association and cognitive areas of the cortex, and may obtain emotional associations from non-auditory subcortical structures such as the limbic system. The complexity of auditory processing is substantial, driven by the many aspects

---

* Correspondence: Allen F. Ryan, Ph.D., University of California, San Diego, 9500 Gilman Drive #0666, La Jolla, CA 92093 ; Phone: 01-858-534-4594; Fax: 01-858-534-5319 (fax); Email: afryan@ucsd.edu

of acoustic signals that are encoded by the system, and by the sheer numbers of neurons and synaptic connections involved. This complexity is increased by the ability of the system to adapt to changing circumstances with both short- and long-term plasticity. Such plasticity is an important component of normal auditory function, but can also be a compensatory response to damage. In addition, plasticity can contribute to auditory disease, or be associated with rehabilitation. Appreciating this damage and treatment-related plasticity requires an understanding of how the normal central auditory system encodes acoustic stimuli, and how this coding may vary depending upon the demands that are placed upon the system.

The human brain is estimated to contain approximately 50-100 billion neurons, most of which are cerebellar granule cells. In the central auditory pathway, 1-2 million subcortical auditory neurons provide input to about 100 million auditory cortical neurons. Since neurons in the brain average one thousand synapses each (Williams and Herrup, 1988), the central auditory system probably contains approximately 100 billion synapses. The increasing numbers of neurons and synapses within the central auditory system provide the basis for extensive processing of auditory stimuli as signals ascend the pathway, with the interplay of excitatory and inhibitory synaptic activity shaping the purely excitatory input that originally derives from hair cells. The synapses also provide the substrate for a high degree of auditory neural plasticity. This plasticity is a normal part of the physiology of the system, which has a remarkable ability to adapt its physiology to match the demands of the acoustic environment and changing circumstances.

This chapter will review our current knowledge of central auditory physiology, including the ability of the normal system to modify its responses, both in the short and long term, based on stimulus context and attention.

Central Auditory Processing Strategies

All of the qualities of sound that we perceive are encoded by the neurons of the cochlear and the central auditory system. Physiological recordings from these neurons at various levels of the system have identified the basic mechanisms by which various acoustic properties are encoded. These include strategies for coding stimulus intensity, frequency, temporal pattern and location in space.

Spontaneous Rat

The majority of auditory neurons discharge even in the absence of acoustic stimulation. This spontaneous discharge provides a background of activity that must be exceeded before evoked activity can influence the neuron. In addition, spontaneous firing can be decreased by inhibitory stimulation, providing an additional mode of evoked changes in neural activity that can be detected and interpreted by the system.

Intensity Coding

The intensity of sounds is encoded by individual neurons primarily as a function of their discharge rate. In the VIIIth nerve, neurons respond very simply to increases in stimulus intensity. Once the threshold of an individual neuron is reached, discharge rate increases above the spontaneous rate in a monotonic manner (that is, without decreasing), until a maximum discharge rate is achieved. Additional increases in intensity thereafter have relatively little effect upon discharge rate. Each individual VIIIth nerve neuron has a dynamic range of about 20 dB. However, a much wider range of intensity is encoded by the activation of neurons with different thresholds, since thresholds of VIIIth nerve fibers vary from approximately 0 to 60 dB SPL (e.g. Chatterjee and Zwislocki, 1998). At any individual frequency region of the nerve, the rage of intensity that can be encoded is thus increased to approximately 80 dB. However, with increased intensity neurons from adjacent frequency regions are recruited. This provides additional range to VIIIth nerve intensity coding.

At higher levels of the system, neural processing provides for neurons which can respond across a wider range of intensity, and with input-output functions that are more complex than those of VIIIth nerve fibers. Inhibitory influences can extend the dynamic range well in excess of 20 dB. Moreover, the intensity functions of central auditory neurons are often non-monotonic, in that discharge rate can increase or decrease in a complex manner, as intensity increases and recruits additional excitatory and inhibitory inputs. The simplest nonmonotonic function occurs when increasing intensity recruits primarily inhibitory inputs, which results in a "best intensity" function in which the neuron's discharge increases to a maximum at a particular intensity, above which discharge is reduced.

Alternatively, within the central auditory pathway neurons may be dominated primarily by inhibitory inputs. In such cases the neurons will respond with decreased firing, below their spontaneous rate, which depends upon intensity. Finally, central auditory neurons may respond with different temporal patterns to different intensities, for example responding only to the onset of an acoustic signal at low intensity, and to the entire signal at higher intensity, or vise versa (e.g. Ryan and Miller, 1977).

An addition mode of intensity encoding is temporal in nature. As signal intensity increases, the temporal link between stimulus and signal increases, decreasing signal latency, increasing the relationship of neural discharge to stimulus phase, and increasing the inter-correlation of discharge spike timing, especially for complex stimuli (Cariani and Delgutte, 1996).

Frequency Coding

In the VIIIth nerve, frequency is encoded tonotopically, by the location of the hair cells from which the neuron receives synaptic input. In this case, the discharge of each fibers is shaped by the pattern of basilar membrane vibration at that location, which in turn is sharpened by the activity of prestin in the outer hair cells at low stimulus intensities. Low-frequency fibers are located in the center of the VIIIth nerve, and progressively higher frequency fibers are added to the surface of the nerve as it passes along the modiolus. This tonotopic or cochleotopic organization is preserved at leach level of the central auditory pathway by the strict projection of axons from one location in the tonotopic field of a given auditory nucleus to the corresponding location in higher nuclei. This organization results in the tuning curves that can be recorded from most individual auditory neurons at all levels of the system, by varying the frequency and intensity of pure tone stimulation.

The tuning curves of VIIIth nerve fibers are entirely excitatory. However, the addition of inhibitory neurons and synapses results in additional complexity in central auditory neurons. It often adds an inhibitory surround to excitation elicited by a preferred frequency (e.g. Young and Brownell, 1976), or can result in purely inhibitory tuning curves. An additional feature of central neurons is summation of inputs from different frequency regions. This can result in tuning curves that are broader than those determined by basilar membrane motion, or even units that respond independently of stimulus frequency.

In addition to spatial frequency coding, VIIIth nerve and higher auditory neurons may also discharge in synchrony with the phase of a stimulus, a process known as phase-locking or frequency following (e.g. Chatterjee and Zwislocki, 1997). Phase-locking operates only at relatively low frequencies. In the auditory nerve, fibers can exhibit at least some degree of phase-locking up to about 5 kHz. Of course, because of their refractory periods individual neurons cannot fire at rates above approximately 500 Hz. However, at higher frequencies they respond to a fraction of the cycles of the tone, at the same phase. By assessing input from many neurons firing in phase with the stimulus, the system as a whole can represent the original signal. At successively higher centers of the central auditory pathway, the upper limits of phase locking decreases, to approximately 1 kHz in the inferior colliculus (Liu et al., 2006) and to 250 Hz in auditory cortex (Wallace et al., 2002). However, this form of frequency coding is particularly important for the encoding of vowel formants in speech (Cariani and Delgutte, 1996).

Temporal Coding

Beyond frequency, the temporal features of an acoustic stimulus include onset, duration, offset and envelope variation. In the VIIIth nerve, these features are approximated in individual fibers by the envelope of neuronal discharge rate above spontaneous activity, with the exception of initial adaptation. Auditory nerve fiber adaptation occurs when the discharge elicited by the onset of a stimulus drops for the first several msec to reach a steady state. Otherwise, neurons follow the envelope of the signal within the constraints of their intensity and frequency responses (e.g. Kiang et al., 1970).

At higher centers, the responses of neurons to temporal variation in an acoustic signal are extensively shaped by neural processing. This can be illustrated by the temporal pattern of the response to a simple tone burst. VIIIth nerve fibers responses displaying only adaptation respond with a "primarlylike" pattern. In the cochlear nucleus some neurons exhibit a similar response, especially those spherical anteroventral nucleus cells dominated by very large synapses from VIIIth nerve fibers, synapses known as endbulbs of Held. However, for other cochlear nucleus cells, input from inhibitory interneurons produces temporal responses consisting of a pause after an initial burst of activity ("pauser"), or bursts of discharge separated by inhibitory intervals ("chopper"), only a single burst of activity ("onset") or by initial inhibition followed by excitation ("buildup") (e.g. Young and Brownell, 1976). Especially at higher levels of the system, even more complex patterns of activity are observed, including "offset" neurons that discharge only when a stimulus terminates, "onset-offset" neurons, and many complex patterns (e.g. Ryan et al., 1984).

Another example of higher auditory temporal processing is provided by the encoding of amplitude modulations in a continuous acoustic signal. At lower levels of the auditory system, neuronal discharge follows the envelope of an amplitude-modulated signal as described above. However, as one ascends the central pathway envelope following decreases, to be replaced by neurons that appear to be "tuned" to particular envelope modulation frequencies (Joris et al., 2004). Thus temporal modulation of signals to some extent becomes encoded as a category in higher centers, rather than as a modulation of spike frequency. This may be because amplitude modulation of signals is often a biologically important feature of sounds.

Sound Localization

The location of sound in space is detected by the central auditory system with considerable accuracy. This is accomplished by comparing the level and timing of neural activity that derives from the two cochleae. Obviously, interaural differences in the intensity and timing of acoustic signals are not encoded in the VIIIth nerve or the cochlear nuclei, since these structures receive almost all of their inputs from a single ear. The neurons of the superior olivary complex, and especially of the medial nucleus of the trapezoid body (MNTB), the medial nucleus of the superior olive (MSO) and the lateral nucleus of the superior olive (LSO) are the first central neurons to receive substantial inputs from both cochleas. Moreover, certain neurons within the olivary nuclei are specialized to compare inputs from the two cochleas, since they possess two dendritic trees that are innervated by fibers that receive inputs from the opposite ears.

Olivary complex neurons appear to evaluate stimulus location via two mechanisms. For high frequency stimuli, head shadowing can produce differences in the intensity of acoustic stimuli that arrive at the two ears if the source is off of the midline. Thus for frequencies above approximately 5 kHz, neurons compare the relative intensity of signals originating from the two ears, as an interaural intensity difference. This mechanism is limited to high frequencies, since stimuli below about 1.5 kHz pass easily around the head, without creating an acoustic shadow. However, as noted above, the phase of low frequency stimuli is encoded by auditory neurons. This allows auditory neurons to compare the arrival time of two signals between the two ears, as an interaural delay.

These two strategies of the central auditory are to some extent segregated anatomically. Low stimulus frequencies are over-represented in the MSO, while high frequencies are over-represented in the LSO (McAlpine, 2005). Neurons recorded in the MSO are low frequency in nature and are highly sensitive to interaural phase and arrival time differences, showing substantial changes in discharge are as these are varied (e.g. Yin and Chan, 1990). In the LSO, neurons receive excitatory inputs from the ipsilateral ear and inhibitory inputs from the contralateral ear. Interaural intensity differences that favor the ipsilateral ear are thus highly excitatory, while those that favor the contralateral ear will suppress discharge. For each neuron, there is a particular interaural intensity difference at which discharge is completely inhibited, and this difference varies for each neuron. This point of minimal discharge, which is the basis for localization of sounds by intensity differences, is thought to be determined by the unique thresholds of inhibition and excitation and the unique latency differences for the opposing inputs to each cell (Park et al., 1997).

Information on sound localization is integrated and additional binaural processing occurs as activity ascends the central auditory pathway (e.g. Moore, 1991). The effect of this processing is to produce cortical neurons with one or more preferred locations in space. That is, the discharge of the neuron is maximal when the stimulus is at a particular location, and lower at other orientations. However, there is evidence that sound localization at the cortical level is localized in areas caudal to primary auditory cortex, rather than in A1 (Recanzone, 2000).

Complex Stimuli

The stimuli most frequently used to study auditory stimuli are kept deliberately simple in order to eliminate extraneous variables. However, these stimuli have the disadvantage that they are of relatively little biological relevance. If fact, the central auditory system of most organisms, humans included, are specialized to perceive stimuli that are of importance. One of the most extreme examples of this is the bat, which is specialized to perceive echos of its own vocalizations from the bodies of flying insects. However, virtually all organisms are specialized to perceive sounds that are important for communication amongst individuals.

For example, Portfors et al. (2009) found that many neurons in the inferior colliculus of mice respond strongly to species-specific vocalizations, even if the frequencies of the calls are outside of the neurons' tuning curves measured with pure tones. This produces a significant over-representation of these calls relative to simple stimuli. This result indicates that the encoding of communication signals occurs by processes that cannot be easily predicted by the standard auditory coding strategies that we typically recognize.

Suta et al. (2008) further evaluated responses to species calls in the guinea pig, by comparing inferior colliculus single unit responses to calls played forward versus backward. Forward calls elicited significantly greater discharge rates than time-reversed calls. Moreover, the neural processing of the forward call could not be predicted purely based on its spectral or temporal content. Discharge rates are not the only manner in which biologically relevant stimuli are encoded. Huetz et al. (2009) examined the response of auditory thalamic and cortical neurons to species-specific calls. They found that even neurons for which there was little or no increase in discharge rate displayed significant changes in discharge timing as revealed by spike-timing reliability analysis.

It has also been suggested that the human auditory system is similarly organized to respond to our own communication signals. For example, PET has been used to demonstrate that forward speech produces activation of left anterior superior temporal gyrus, while backward speech does not (Wong et al., 2002). This asymmetry does not appear to depend upon experience. Using optical topographic assessment of blood flow, Pena et al. (2003) found that the left temporal cortical responses of newborn infants to forward speech were significantly more robust than those to backward speech, even if the speech stimuli used were not from the native language of their parents. Right hemisphere responses did not show a similar disparity. These results suggest that the processing of speech signals in humans is inherently different from those of non-speech stimuli, even ones with similar spectral and temporal characteristics. Thus the central auditory system of the human, like thos of toher species, may be specifically adapted for the perception of acoustic stimuli with characteristics similar to human speech.

Variation in the Physiology of the Normal Central Auditory Pathway

The coding characteristics of auditory neurons described above are often treated as invariant properties of the auditory neurons. However, this impression is an artifact of the experimental procedures that are most often used to evaluate them. This includes the use of extremely simplified acoustic environments, often consisting of short bursts at a single stimulus frequency. In addition, most neurophysiological studies are conducted in anesthetized animals, which can severely alter the responses of neurons. In addition, almost all laboratory investigations of central physiology use stimuli that are of no relevance to the animal being studied, and with which the animals have had no previous experience.

In order to appreciate central auditory physiology as it functions during perception, it is important to understand the influence of these factors. This is especially important since studies that circumvent these variables have shown that the intrinsic responses of central auditory neurons can vary extensively, and that central auditory response properties can be modulated throughout the central auditory system by activity that originates from higher levels of the auditory system or from non-auditory neural centers. These factors play a significant role in auditory attention and in learned processing of auditory stimuli.

Anesthesia

Anesthetics, by their nature, induce a profound depression of the central nervous system, often by enhancing activity at classes of inhibitory synapses or by depressing activity at excitatory synapses. Thus central auditory responses observed in anesthetized animals represent this altered state of the system. The influence of anesthetics is most obvious at higher levels of the central auditory pathway. In fact, early studies of cortex in anesthetized animals found that it was rather difficult to evoke consistent activity in cortical neurons using acoustic stimuli that were quite effective in lower auditory nuclei (e.g. Erulkar et al., 1956; Whitfield, 1967). Only when neural responses began to be recorded from unanesthetized preparations did robust responses of auditory cortical neurons emerge (e.g. Miller et al. 1972). Anesthetics influence not only the responsiveness but also the basic response properties of cortical neurons. Gaese and Oswald (2001) found that anesthesia led to increased sharpness of tuning curves for in the majority of neurons in the auditory cortex of guinea pigs. Feng et al. (2009) observed a loss of ability of cortical neurons to follow acoustic envelope variations under anesthesia, suggesting a degradation of temporal coding.

While the neurons of the auditory cortex may be the most sensitive, the activity of neurons in the lower levels of the central auditory system can also be influenced by anesthetics. Torterolo et al. (2002) found that pentobarbital, which mimics the effects of the inhibitory neurotransmitter GABA at $GABA_A$ receptors, reduced spontaneous and evoked firing rates, reduced the duration of excitatory responses and enhanced post-excitatory suppression of inferior colliculus neurons. Astl et al. (1996) also noted changes in response patterns, with a preponderance of onset units under pentobarbital anesthesia.

Wang et al. (1987) assessed the effects of pentobarbital anesthesia on evoked central auditory metabolic activity, using a deoxyglucose uptake assay which reflects both discharge and synaptic activity. They noted a profound depression of evoked neural activity in the dorsal nucleus of the lateral lemniscus and all higher auditory centers, but enhanced auditory evoked activity in the ventral nucleus of the lateral lemniscus and all lower centers. Ketamine, which acts by blocking excitatory NMDA receptors, had a similar effect.

Anesthesia has also been found to influence central auditory physiology in humans. Schwender et al. (1995) recorded auditory brainstem response (ABR) and cortically generated middle latency auditory evoked potentials (MLAEPs) prior to and during general anesthesia in surgical patients. They found modest increases in the latency of ABR wave V, but more3 dramatic latency increases for cortical potentials. They also noted significant decreases in the amplitude of MLAEPs.

These data indicate that the physiology of the auditory system studied in anesthetized animals and humans is more heavily weighted toward inhibition. In the awake animal and human, excitatory responses are likely to be significantly more important in shaping the responses of central auditory neurons.

Development

The responses of the central auditory pathway also change markedly during development. This is particular relevant for humans, for whom the maturation of the central nervous system requires many years. For example, while the anatomical development of the human brainstem auditory nuclei is essentially complete at age two, Johnson et al. (2008) noted very significant improvements in frequency and temporal representation in auditory brainstem responses, during the period of maturation from infancy into adolescence. Moreover, experience can alter the patterns of auditory processing during the developmental period. For example, Yu et al. (2007) found that mice, exposed to two tones at moderate level during development, showed very strong representation of these two frequencies in the adult cortex, when compared to normally reared mice. This type of plasticity fits well with the idea of critical periods during development, during which the response of a system can change in response to the environment early in development, but loses this plasticity as the system matures.

The ability of humans to acquire language is well known to be limited by an early critical period. It has been extensively documented that individuals who are prelingually deaf have great difficulty in processing acoustic signals comprehending speech due to lack of experience early in life, even if the function of the central auditory pathway is restored through a CI (e.g. Sharma and Dorman, 2006). Although difficulties in communication are thought to be limited by critical periods in the development of speech and language centers (e.g. Amunts et al., 2003), the central auditory system also has critical periods for processing speech signals. Højen and Flege (2006) found that the auditory processing of English vowel formants by those who learned English as a second language early in life differed from that of individuals who learned the language later in life. Thus the auditory processing of speech signals is subject to a critical developmental period of enhanced central auditory plasticity.

However, the central auditory system can also exhibit plasticity in the normal adult, and the degree of this plasticity can be profound.

Attention

The central auditory system is remarkable for its ability to extract information of relevance from a background of competing auditory stimuli. This process depends upon extraction of relevant features from the acoustic environment, and upon the suppression of irrelevant signals. This process is known to be associated with changes in the response properties of auditory neurons. For example, Miller et al. (1972) found that the responses of auditory cortical neurons in awake animals that were attending to a stimulus in a behavioral task were significantly enhanced compared to those recorded when the animal was passively listening. The involvement of the cortex in plasticity associated with attention is not surprising, and is consistent with models of a "thalamic gate" operating to limit the transmission of sensory information from subcortical sensory pathways into the cortex (Scheibel and Scheibel, 1966; Skinner and Yingling, 1977; Yingling and Skinner, 1977).

Thalamic gate models predict that the responses of auditory neurons in nuclei below the level of the medial geniculate nucleus would be less sensitive to attentional state than would cortical neurons. However, Ryan and Miller (1977) found that the responses of neurons in the inferior colliculus, a midbrain structure, were also highly sensitive to attention. They observed substantial changes in response properties between attending to a stimulus in a reaction time task as compared to passive listening. For example, a neuron that responded with a burst of firing to both the onset and the offset of a stimulus delivered passively responded only to the onset when the animal was attending. Moreover, similar results were later obtained from auditory neurons in the brainstem, even at the level of the cochlear nucleus (Ryan et al., 1984). These included changes in latency, discharge, temporal pattern and intensity functions. These observations indicate that the responses of neurons can be significantly altered by cortical descending inputs, throughout the central auditory pathway. These changes alter central auditory processing in order to extract relevant information from auditory stimuli against a background of irrelevant stimuli.

It is impossible to reproduce in humans the precision of single unit studies that have demonstrated attentional changes in the central auditory system of animals. Evoked potentials that sum the responses of vast numbers of cells can detect only global changes in central auditory processing. However, despite the limitations, changes in central auditory responses related to attention have also been noted in humans. Many studies have demonstrated that auditory cortical potentials can be influenced by selective attention to a stimulus (e.g. Woldorff et al., 1987, Näätänen and Teder, 1991).

There may be more than one mode by which attention influences auditory cortex. Ahlo (1992) found that the distribution of changes in auditory cortical evoked potential produced by attention to a visual stimulus was different from the distribution seen when the subject was attending to a different auditory stimulus. Woldorff and Hillyard (1991) evaluated auditory evoked potentials generated tones of different frequencies delivered to the opposite ears, when subjects were attending to one ear or the other. They noted consistent changes in the evoked responses, depending upon attention, as early as 20 msec after stimulus onset.

However, some evidence suggests that attention-related changes occur for lower level central auditory processing of humans, as well. While most studies of auditory brainstem evoked responses (ABRs) have failed to detect changes with selective attention (see Michie et al. (1996) for a review), a few investigators have observed altered potentials. For example, Lukas (1981) compared the effects of visual or auditory attention on the ABR, and found that only attention to an auditory task influenced the potentials. Evaluating a different mechanism of coding, Galbraith et al. (2003) assessed the brainstem evoked frequency following response and found a significant enhancement of amplitude associated with attention. An intriguing observation was made by Giard et al. (1994) who reported small (0.5 dB) but consistent enhancement of evoked otoacoustic emissions related to attention. Maison et al., (2001) obtained evidence that attention to an auditory signal in one ear produced a frequency-specific enhancement of otoacoustic emissions in the opposite ear. The results of these studies suggest that descending inputs related to attention can influence even the responses of the inner ear.

Plasticity of auditory processing related to attentional state is transient, occurring over the course of seconds or minutes, and lasting only as long as attention is focused. These changes are presumably mediated by alterations in the balance of excitatory and inhibitory synaptic inputs to auditory neurons, which can be modulated by descending inputs from auditory and non-auditory structures. Such changes in excitatory/inhibitory balance can sometimes be directly inferred from the responses of individual central auditory neurons. For example, reaction time performance can be associated with a period of late suppression of discharge that occurs approximately 150 msec before the behavioral response in some neurons, consistent with a transient period of descending inhibition of the neuron after stimulus detection. Once the descending inputs are removed or altered, however, the neurons return to their previous auditory processing state. Descending cortical effects can be modeled by the electrical stimulation of auditory cortex in animals. Yan and Ehret (2001) stimulated primary auditory cortex in the mouse, and recorded frequency tuning in the inferior colliculus. They found that frequency tuning in the midbrain shifted towards the frequency at the locus of cortical stimulation, demonstrating that auditory cortex can reorganize a basic feature of subcortical auditory processing.

Transient biochemical or molecular changes within a neuron ("intrinsic plasticity") may also be involved in some types of short-term central auditory plasticity (Hennig et al., 2008).

Conclusions

The central auditory system employs a variety of strategies to encode the features of acoustic stimuli. These strategies have been documented in many studies of the responses of neurons in the pathway to sound, and we therefore understand the basic mechanisms by which features of a stimulus are encoded, including loudness, frequency, temporal pattern and position in space. However, it is important to note that most such studies have been accomplished using artificial stimuli that are of little relevance, and in anesthetized animals. These studies seriously underestimate the complexity of responses to sound by the central auditory pathway. They also ignore responses to stimuli that are of particular relevance to the organism. This relevance can dramatically alter central coding. By understanding these more complex features of auditory physiology we can better appreciate the mechanisms that underlie the plasticity of the system to experience, when it is challenged by damage, or how plasticity may influence therapy.

Acknowledgments

Supported by the Research Service of the US Veterans Administration and NIH/NIDCD grant DC00139.

References

Alho, K. Selective attention in auditory processing as reflected by event-related brain potentials. *Psychophysiology.* 1992, 29 :247-263.

Amunts, K; Schleicher, A; Ditterich, A; Zilles, K. Broca's region: cytoarchitectonic asymmetry and developmental changes. *J Comp Neurol.* 2003, 465: 72-89.

Astl, J; Popelár, J; Kvasnák, E; Syka, J. Comparison of response properties of neurons in the inferior colliculus of guinea pigs under different anesthetics. *Audiology.* 1996, 35 :335-345.

Cariani, PA; Delgutte, B. Neural correlates of the pitch of complex tones. I. Pitch and pitch salience. *J Neurophysiol.* 1996, 76 :1698-1716.

Chatterjee, M; Zwislocki, JJ. Cochlear mechanisms of frequency and intensity coding. I. The place code for pitch. *Hear Res.* 1997, 111: 65-75.

Chatterjee, M; Zwislocki, JJ. Cochlear mechanisms of frequency and intensity coding. II. Dynamic range and the code for loudness. *Hear Res.* 1998, 124 :170-181.

Erulkar, SD; Rose, JE; Davies, PW. Single unit activity in the auditory cortex of the cat. *Bull Johns Hopkins Hosp.* 1956, 99: 55-86.

Feng, Y; Yin, S; Wang, J. Cortical responses to amplitude modulation in guinea pigs and the effects of general anesthesia by pentobarbital. *Hear Res.* 2009, 247 :40-46.

Gaese, BH; Ostwald, J. Anesthesia changes frequency tuning of neurons in the rat primary auditory cortex. *J Neurophysiol.* 2001, 86 :1062-1066.

Galbraith, GC; Olfman, DM; Huffman, TM. Selective attention affects human brain stem frequency-following response. *Neuroreport* 2003, 14: 735-738.

Giard, MH; Collet, L; Bouchet, P; Pernier, J. Auditory selective attention in the human cochlea. *Brain Res.* 1994, 633 :353-356.

Hennig, MH; Postlethwaite, M; Forsythe, ID; Graham, BP. Interactions between multiple sources of short-term plasticity during evoked and spontaneous activity at the rat calyx of Held. *J Physiol.* 2008, 586 :3129-46.

Højen, A; Flege, JE. Early learners' discrimination of second-language vowels. *J Acoust Soc Am.* 2006, 119 :3072-3084.

Huetz, C; Philibert, B; Edeline, JM. A spike-timing code for discriminating conspecific vocalizations in the thalamocortical system of anesthetized and awake guinea pigs. *J Neurosci.* 2009, 29 :334-350.

Irvine, DR; Rajan, R; Smith, S. Effects of restricted cochlear lesions in adult cats on the frequency organization of the inferior colliculus. *J Comp Neurol.* 2003, 467 :354-374.

Johnson, KL; Nicol, T; Zecker, SG; Kraus, N. Developmental plasticity in the human auditory brainstem. *J Neurosci.* 2008, 28 :4000-4007.

Joris, PX; Schreiner, CE; Rees, A. Neural processing of amplitude-modulated sounds. *Physiol Rev.* 2004, 84 :541-577.

Kiang, NY; Moxon, EC; Levine, RA. Auditory-nerve activity in cats with normal and abnormal cochleas. In: Sensorineural hearing loss. *Ciba Found Symp.* 1970, :241-273.

Liu, LF; Palmer, AR; Wallace, MN. Phase-locked responses to pure tones in the inferior colliculus. *J Neurophysiol.* 2006, 95 :1926-1935.

Lukas JH. The role of efferent inhibition *Int J Neurosci.* 1981;12(2):137-45.

Maison S, Micheyl C, Collet L. Influence of focused auditory attention on cochlear activity in humans. *Psychophysiol.* 2001 Jan;38(1):35-40.

McAlpine, D. Creating a sense of auditory space. *J Physiol.* 2005, 566 :21-28.

Michie, PT; LePage, EL; Solowij, N; Haller, M; Terry, L. Evoked otoacoustic emissions and auditory selective attention. *Hear Res.* 1996, 98 :54-67.

Miller, J; Sutton, D; Pfingst, B; Ryan, AF; Beaton, R; Gourevitch, G. Single cell activity in the auditory cortex of Rhesus monkeys: Behavioral dependency. *Science* 1972, :449-451.

Moore, DR. Anatomy and physiology of binaural hearing. *Audiology.* 1991, 30 :125-134.

Näätänen, R; Teder, W. Attention effects on the auditory event-related potential. *Acta Otolaryngol Suppl.* 1991, 491 :161-166.

Park, TJ; Monsivais, P; Pollak, GD. Processing of interaural intensity differences in the LSO: role of interaural threshold differences. *J Neurophysiol.* 1997, 77 :2863-2878.

Portfors, CV; Roberts, PD; Jonson, K. Over-representation of species-specific vocalizations in the awake mouse inferior colliculus. *Neuroscience.* 2009, 162 :486-500.

Recanzone, GH. Spatial processing in the auditory cortex of the macaque monkey. *Proc Natl Acad Sci U S A.* 2000, 97 :11829-11835.

Ryan, A; Miller J. Effect of behavioural performance on single unit firing patterns in the inferior colliculus of the Rhesus monkey. *J Neurophysiol* 1977, 40: 943-956.

Ryan, AF; Miller, J; Pfingst, BE; Martin, GK. Effects of reaction time performance upon single-unit discharge in the central auditory pathway of the Rhesus monkey. *J Neurosci* 1984, 4: 298-308.

Scheibel, ME; Scheibel, AB. The organization of the nucleus reticularis thalami: a Golgi study. *Brain Res.* 1966, 1 :43-62.

Schwender D, Weninger E, Daunderer M, Klasing S, Pöppel E, Peter K. Anesthesia with increasing doses of sufentanil and midlatency auditory evoked potentials *Anesth Analg.* 1995 Mar;80(3):499-505.

Sharma, A; Dorman, MF. Central auditory development in children with cochlear implants: clinical implications. *Adv Otorhinolaryngol.* 2006, 64 :66-88.

Skinner, JE; Yingling, CD. Reconsideration of the cerebral mechanisms underlying selective attention and slow potential shifts. In Desmedt JE, (Ed) *Attention, voluntary contraction and event-related cerebral potentials. Progress in clinical neurophysiology,* Vol 1, pp 30-69. Basel: Karger, 1977.

Suta, D; Popelár, J; Syka, J. Coding of communication calls in the subcortical and cortical structures of the auditory system. *Physiol Res.* 2008, 3 :S149-159.

Torterolo, P; Falconi, A; Morales-Cobas, G; Velluti, RA. Inferior colliculus unitary activity in wakefulness, sleep and under barbiturates. *Brain Res.* 2002, 935 :9-15.

Wallace, MN; Shackleton, TM; Palmer, AR. Phase-locked responses to pure tones in the primary auditory cortex. *Hear Res.* 2002, 172 :160-171.

Wang, ZX; Ryan, AF; Woolf, N. Pentobarbital and ketamine on alter 2-deoxyglucose uptake patterns in the central auditory system of the gerbil. *Hear Res* 1987, 27: 145-155.

Whitfield IC. Coding in the auditory nervous system *Nature.* 1967 Feb 25;213(5078):756-60.

Williams, RW; Herrup, K. The control of neuron number. *Ann Rev Neurosci* 1988, 11: 423–453.

Woldorff, M; Hansen, JC; Hillyard, SA. Evidence for effects of selective attention in the mid-latency range of the human auditory event-related potential. *Electroencephalogr Clin Neurophysiol Suppl.* 1987, 40 :146-154.

Woldorff, MG; Hillyard, SA. Modulation of early auditory processing during selective listening to rapidly presented tones. *Electroencephalogr Clin Neurophysiol.* 1991, 79 :170-191.

Wong, D; Pisoni, DB; Learn, J; Gandour, JT; Miyamoto, RT; Hutchins, GD. PET imaging of differential cortical activation by monaural speech and nonspeech stimuli. *Hear Res.* 2002, 166 :9-23.

Yan, J; Ehret, G. Corticofugal reorganization of the midbrain tonotopic map in mice. *Neuroreport.* 2001, 12 :3313-3316.

Yin, TC; Chan, JC. Interaural time sensitivity in medial superior olive of cat. *J Neurophysiol* 1990, 64: 465–488.

Yingling, CD; Skinner, JE. *Gating of Thalamic Input to Cerebral Cortex by Nucleus Reticularis Thalami* vol. 1, Karger, Basel, 1977.

Young, ED; Brownell, WE. Responses to tones and noise of single cells in dorsal cochlear nucleus of unanesthetized cats. *J Neurophysiol.* 1976, 39 :282-300.

Yu, X; Sanes, DH; Aristizabal, O; Wadghiri, YZ; Turnbull, DH. Large-scale reorganization of the tonotopic map in mouse auditory midbrain revealed by MRI. *Proc Natl Acad Sci U S A.* 2007, 104 :12193-12198.

In: Neuroplasticity in the Auditory Brainstem   ISBN 978-1-61761-949-6
Editor: Angelo Salami, pp. 31- 44   © 2011 Nova Science Publishers, Inc.

Chapter III

Neurobiology of Age Related Hearing Loss

L. Guastini, V. Santomauro, M. Dellepiane, R. Mora, B. Crippa, A. Salami

ENT Department, University of Genoa, Italy

Abstract

The deterioration of hearing function, particularly at high frequencies, is a process that inevitably accompanies aging in humans as well as in other mammals. The etiology of the disease remains unknown, although, as in other age related diseases, histopathological abnormalities can be identified. The knowledge of the neurobiological mechanisms may be useful to understand the pathophysiology of presbycusis and thus define new therapeutic strategies.

Somatic mitochondrial DNA (mtDNA) deletions have been associated with the process of aging in many postmitotic tissues. The cochlear tissues are known to contain an abundance of mitochondria, and this observation has prompted a search for mtDNA deletions in the cochlea. The presence of the common deletion (CD) has been reported in the mtDNA isolated from cochlear tissues of individuals with presbycusis. The function of the cochlea is to convert an acoustic signal into an electrochemical stimulus, which is then transmitted to the central nervous system. Cochlea tissue like muscle, heart, and brain tissues has an abundance of mitochondria and is expected to be heavily dependent on functional mitochondria. The role of mtDNA mutations in presbycusis and aging has been investigated: an high frequency of mtDNA point mutations has been reported in temporal bones of individuals with presbycusis. The consequence of mtDNA mutations is a deficit in energy metabolism and their presence may trigger apoptosis; mtDNA mutations only become physiologically important when a threshold level is exceeded. This level may vary between tissues based on the energy metabolism required for function.

Mitochondrial dysfunction plays a role in the pathogenesis of presbycusis, and bioenergetics agents such as creatine, coenzyme Q10, or nicotinamide may be neuroprotective in presbycusis.

Coenzyme Q10 inhibits lipid peroxidation by either scavenging free radicals directly or by reducing a-tocopheroxyl radical to a-tocopherol. Coenzyme Q10 protects membrane proteins against oxidation. Coenzyme Q10 also inhibits DNA oxidation in rat liver mitochondria and inhibits DNA strand breaks in human lymphocytes. In the cochlea, coenzyme Q10 presumably prevents lipid oxidation, protein oxidation, and DNA damage.

The findings illustrated in this chapter represent the experimental basis for the development of a new therapies in the treatment of presbycusis, addressed to prevent lipid peroxidation and mitochondrial damage.

Introduction

There are many different sensory systems. The somatic sensory system mediates the sense of touch and the proprioceptive division relays information about internal parts of the body. The auditory system provides hearing, located in the same area is the vestibular system, which provides a sense a balance. The olfactory system and the gustatory system mediate the sense of smell and taste.

Each system has a specific receptor: vision transduction requires photoreceptors; audition, mechanoreceptors; taste and smell, chemoreceptors, and the touch system uses mechanoreceptors, thermoreceptors and nociceptors (pain receptors).

The conversion of outside signals to chemical signals in the brain is referred to as transduction, and sensory transduction in the various systems shares a few characteristics. Sensory receptors (neurons, in the somatic sensory and olfactory systems, and epithelial cells in the visual, auditory, gustatory systems) synapse on an interneuron that relays signals to the brain. Each one of these modalities has its own pathway, and a relay through the subnuclei of the thalamus, and eventually terminate in a specific area of the cortex.

Perceptions can vary in four ways: modality (auditory, visual, etc.), intensity, duration and location. Variations in sensation are encoded in variations in action potentials.

The role of the auditory system in mammals is to inform the subject about the acoustical environment and about the presence of species-specific acoustical communication signals. In humans, the latter function is dominant since one of the specific features of humans is the ability to learn and use language.

In mammals, the loss of hearing receptors at an early postnatal age results in plastic changes in the central auditory system similarly like in the visual and somatosensory systems [1]. In mammals, in contrast to other vertebrates, the hair cells in the cochlea do not regenerate and the plastic processes in the central auditory system may be different from other vertebrates: the loss of hearing function may not necessarily be complete, but even a partial decline in the number of inner ear receptors results in a limitation of hearing function in humans, especially in the intelligibility of speech [1]. The deterioration of hearing function, particularly at high frequencies, is a process that inevitably accompanies aging in humans as well as in other mammals [1].

The etiology of the disease remains unknown, although, as in other age related diseases, histopathological abnormalities can be identified. These abnormalities include degenerative changes in the cochlea, including the spiral ganglion cells, stria vascularis, inner hair cells, and outer hair cells [2]. For these reasons knowledge of the neurobiological mechanisms may be useful to understand the pathophysiology of presbycusis and thus define new therapeutic strategies.

Neurobiology

The dominant component of presbycusis is the gradual degeneration of hair cells mainly in the basal part of the cochlea; however, its central component is usually based on sclerotic processes in the brain. It is the aim of contemporary research to recognize the compensatory processes that exist in the adult auditory system with the aim of utilizing them for the rehabilitation of hearing function [1].

Several genes that play a role in how our body's cells normally auto-destruct may play a role in age-related hearing loss, according to recent researches several authors know that genetics play some role in such hearing loss, which affects nearly everyone older than 60, as well as many people somewhat younger [3]. But while more than 100 genes are known to play a role in congenital deafness, scientists have yet to pinpoint any gene in humans that plays a role in presbycusis, or age-related hearing loss [3].

The overall age-related loss of hair cells and spiral ganglion cells in the cochlea is of varying magnitude depending on species or strain [3-5]. Evidence that the auditory periphery is clearly affected by age concurs with multiple investigations that show auditory brainstem structures to exhibit substantial deficits in neuronal processing over age in humans [3-5]. In the auditory system presbycusis is associated with specific plastic alterations [3-5]. These plastic alterations are related with several areas of the central nervous system.

Age-related hearing loss is the third most prevalent chronic medical condition among older adults [6]. When accompanied by age-related declines in attentional resources, working memory capacity, and processing speed, one can see the challenge facing many older adults as they attempt to comprehend and remember fast-paced speech in their everyday lives. In addition to missed or incorrectly identified words, diminished hearing may also lead to impoverished, less discriminable memory traces. There is, however, an additional concern: as supported by different authors, successful perception in the face of degraded input may come at the cost of attentional resources that might otherwise be available for encoding what has been heard in memory [6].

Because it could be a problem in the brain, or the problem could rest with any number of cells in the inner ear, age-related hearing loss is a very serious problem for patients, and it's also challenging for scientists who study it. The causes are more complicated than in a condition like Parkinson's disease, where we know exactly which type of cell dies in which part of the brain [7].

In contrast with previous reports that showed a loss of spiral ganglion neurons subsequent to hair cell death [8], other experiences have observed neither hair cell death, nor loss of spiral ganglion neurons [1]. Recent studies have shown a significant and progressive loss in hearing sensitivity in presbycusis: these experiences have highlighted that hearing loss was not generally associated with a severe deterioration of inner ear structure, loss of hair cell phenotype or with a loss of spiral ganglion neurons [1].

This suggests that the hearing loss may be related to an inability of the central nervous system to function adequately in response to an age-altered input from the periphery, as previously proposed by others authors [9,10]. The decline in neuronal plasticity during the adult life span has been proposed to be associated with a reduced level of the effectors of plasticity responses (e.g., BDNF) [1]: the concept of BDNF playing a significant role in the plastic communication events between the peripheral and central nervous system is further supported by the expression of BDNF protein in nerve projections.

Single fibre recordings in the auditory nerves of young and aged gerbils revealed a severe age-related reduction in the activity of low spontaneous rates (low-SR) at characteristic frequencies >6 kHz [11]. Data from a recent study of single auditory nerve fibre recordings in the C57BL/6 mouse, which also shows age-dependent hearing loss, suggest a decreased maximal spontaneous rate among fibres from the high-frequency hearing impaired region [12].

These findings are supported by recent studies indicating that auditory nerve activity plays a critical role in maintaining normal synaptic function at the end bulb of Held, the synapse between auditory nerve fibres and bushy cells in the anterior ventral cochlear nucleus (AVCN), which is the first central auditory relay nucleus [13]. During aging, a significant reduction of release, particularly in the high-frequency areas of synapses at the end bulb of Held in the AVCN was observed [14].

Auditory nerve fibre activity is also the likely input to the crossed-olivocochlear reflex, a reflex that serves an antimasking role in the detection of sounds in a binaural noise field, explaining why reduced activity of auditory nerve may be directly linked to reduced temporal coding observed during presbycusis [15]. The temporal structure of sound has been directly linked to GABAergic inhibition and reduced GABAergic inhibition was also found in the brainstem as a functional neurochemical correlate of age-dependent cochlear or cognitive dysfunction [16]. Again an age-dependent reduction in the release of BDNF at brainstem synapses could be an important factor considering the known effect of BDNF on GABAergic transmission [2].

Reduced BDNF levels in neuritis could thus explain many of the hearing deficits often seen in older individuals, e.g., decreased ability to understand speech in noise, changes in masking level differences and decreased ability to localize sound sources using binaural cues [2].

Because BDFN is a protein belonging to the family of neurotrophins, it's necessary a hint on neurotrophins [17,18].

Neurotrophins

During normal life, up to 80% of the neurons in diverse cell populations within the forming nervous system die. This is thought to be a mechanism that ensures that adequate numbers of neurons establish appropriate innervation densities with effector organs or other neuronal populations. In several instances, the innervation target of a population of neurons has been shown to have a crucial role in regulating the number of surviving neurons. Targets of neuronal innervation produce a limited supply of neurotrophic factors, and competition between neurons responsive to these factors determines which neurons survive [17]. These neurotrophic factors and their receptors direct and regulate proliferation, migration, differentiation, and cell death by acting at different stages in the same or different ways. These factors have been shown to interact with each other directly and indirectly. They may influence different parts of a neuron or glia, through which they may travel considerable distances in time and space [17].

Among them, neurotrophins are a family of proteins important for the normal development and ongoing maintenance of auditory neurons. It is thought that hair cells in the organ of Corti provide the auditory neurons with a continual source of neurotrophins [17].

It is thought that hair cells in the organ of Corti provide the auditory neurons with a continual source of neurotrophins [17]. Interruption to this supply, as a result of damage to the hair cells, is considered a major factor leading to the secondary degeneration of auditory neurons [18]. Although there are a number of different neurotrophins that act throughout the nervous system, it is known that brainderived neurotrophic factor (BDNF) and neurotrophin-3 (NT-3) are essential for auditory neurons to develop and maintain a normal innervation of the inner ear [18].

Over recent years, the intracochlear administration of neurotrophins to prevent and potentially reverse degeneration of auditory neurons following deafening has received much attention. In the adult cochlea, administration of neurotrophins (BDNF and/or NT-3) following deafening was shown to prevent the degeneration of spiral ganglion cells (SGCs) [19], leading to speculation that neurotrophin treatment may present an effective future therapy for protecting the auditory nerve. Neural activity also plays an important role in SGC survival. In vitro studies have demonstrated that depolarization provides trophic support to SGCs during development. In mature animals, the loss of hair cells results in a dramatic reduction of both driven and spontaneous neural activity in SGCs [20].

Excitatory and inhibitory neurotransmitter receptors play key roles in regulating the function and plasticity of the central and peripheral nervous system [21]. Glutamate, γ-amino-butyric acid (GABA) and glycine receptors (GlyR) are known to undergo significant functional changes during critical stages of development both *in vivo* and in vitro [22]. In the central auditory system, there is a profound switch from GABAergic to glycinergic neurotransmission in the lateral superior olivary complex (LSO) during development [23].

Interestingly, the plasticity of this inhibitory synapse is thought to be mediated by brain derived neurotrophic factor (BDNF) and neurotrophic factor 3 (NT-3), two of the most broadly expressed neurotrophic factors (NFs) that bind to tyrosine kinase (Trk) receptors [23].

- BDNF: is a protein that, in humans, is encoded by the *BDNF* gene BDNF is a member of the neurotrophin family of growth factors, which are related to the canonical "Nerve Growth Factor" (NGF). BDNF was the second neurotrophic factor to be characterized after NGF. Neurotrophic factors are found in the brain and the periphery [24].
- BDNF acts on certain neurons of the central nervous system and the peripheral nervous system, helping to support the survival of existing neurons, and encourage the growth and differentiation of new neurons and synapses. BDNF itself is important for long-term memory [24]. Although the vast majority of neurons in the mammalian brain are formed prenatally, parts of the adult brain retain the ability to grow new neurons from neural stem cells in a process known as *neurogenesis*. Neurotrophins are chemicals that help to stimulate and control neurogenesis, BDNF being one of the most active.
- Neurotrophin-3, or NT-3, is a neurotrophic factor, in the NGF-family of neurotrophins. It is a protein growth factor which has activity on certain neurons of the peripheral and central nervous system; it helps to support the survival and differentiation of existing neurons, and encourages the growth and differentiation of new neurons and synapses.
- Previous works suggest that NT3 may play a role in directing migration of neurons and targeting of cochlear axons in the embryonic cochlear nucleus; interestingly, there is a pause in the production of NT3 around birth, when it briefly disappears. When it reappears several days later, presumably it assumes a different role. Because the presence of NT3 in the early stages of synaptogenesis is scanty but becomes abundant with the formation of the definitive synapses, we conclude that this trophic factor very probably does not play a critical role in the early stage of synaptogenesis. We suggest that it plays some role in stabilizing the established structures, for example, the fully formed synapses [25].
- NT-3 was the third neurotrophic factor to be characterized, after NGF and BDNF NT-3 is unique among the neurotrophins in the number of neurons it can potentially stimulate, given its ability to activate two of the receptor tyrosine kinase neurotrophin receptors (TrkC and TrkB). Mice born

without the ability to make NT-3 have loss of proprioceptive and subsets of mechanoreceptive sensory [26].

A role for the neurotrophins neurotrophin 3 (NT3) and brain-derived neurotrophic factor (BDNF) in the normal development and function of the auditory and vestibular systems has long been sought NT3 may be more important for the auditory system, BDNF for the vestibular system [26].

BDNF show the neuroprotective action by reducing the level of 3NP. 3-NP is an irreversible suicide inhibitor of mitochondrial respiration that, upon oxidation by complex II, forms a covalent adduct with a catalytic base arginine in the active site of this enzyme; mitochondrial complex II is believed to be the primary enzyme, in addition to cellular pyridine nucleotide cofactors NADH and NADPH [25]. 3-NP also inhibits lactate dehydrogenase (LDH) [27].

Recent studies show the molecular mechanisms of the neuroprotection induced by BDNF:

- appropriate concentrations (1–5 mM) of GSNO, a slowly releasing NO donor neutralized 3-NP toxicity;
- reduced glutamate evoked apoptosis in hippocampal neurons, trough the activation of ERK1/2, PI3-K, and induction of Bcl-2 proteins.

Mitochondrial Modifications

Cellular energy metabolism occurs in the mitochondria. Mitochondria contain approximately 900 different proteins, 13 of which are coded by the mitochondrial DNA (mtDNA) genome and the remainder coded by nuclear DNA [28]. MtDNA is maternally inherited, and unlike nuclear DNA, each cell contains thousands of mtDNA copies. MtDNA mutations can accumulate in postmitotic cells over time [28]. The functional capacity of mitochondria is dependent on the ratio of mutated genome copies to normal copies within an individual cell: when the ratio exceeds a threshold level, the phenotypic expression of a mutation is observed [28].

This threshold can vary depending on the mutation and cell type. Once the threshold is reached, the cell becomes respiratory deficient. Except for the small noncoding D-loop region (about 1 kilobase [kb]), expression of the whole mitochondrial genome is essential for bioenergetic function as the mtDNA contains no introns. MtDNA mutations can exist as point mutations, nucleotide insertions or deletions, and large deletions. MtDNA deletions are reported to accumulate with age in a variety of tissues [28].

An association between cochlear element degeneration and the severity of hearing loss in individuals with presbycusis has been demonstrated in previous study [29].

Somatic mtDNA deletions have been associated with the process of aging in many postmitotic tissues. The cochlear tissues are known to contain an abundance of mitochondria, and this observation has prompted a search for mtDNA deletions in the cochlea. The presence of the common deletion (CD) has been reported in the mtDNA isolated from cochlear tissues of individuals with presbycusis [30].

The mtDNA deletion most commonly associated with aging is a 4,977–base pair (bp) deletion referred to as the CD. The CD occurs between two 13-bp nucleotide repeat sites, removing approximately 5 kb of mtDNA between the ATP 8 and the ND5 genes. The CD, the genetic defect associated with the Kearns Sayre syndrome, has been detected in heart muscle, brain, skeletal muscle, and other tissues of older individuals [31].

A wide spectrum of diseases is attributed to pathogenic mutations in the mitochondrial genome. The effects of these mutations are more prominent in tissues with high energy demand [31].

The function of the cochlea is to convert an acoustic signal into an electrochemical stimulus, which is then transmitted to the central nervous system. Cochlea tissue like muscle, heart, and brain tissues has an abundance of mitochondria and is expected to be heavily dependent on functional mitochondria. The role of mtDNA mutations in presbycusis and aging has been investigated: an high frequency of mtDNA point mutations has been reported in temporal bones of individuals with presbycusis [32].

A temporal bone study has also demonstrated that the CD is frequently present in cases of presbycusis, less commonly in age matched controls, and rarely in young and middle aged individuals [32].

Recently, different authors have quantified the CD level in cochlear tissue from individuals with presbycusis and demonstrated its association with the severity of hearing loss [2]. The total burden of all mtDNA deletions present in a single cell, however, may be more relevant than the CD level alone with respect to deficits in cellular energy metabolism and as a potential trigger for cell apoptosis [2].

The consequence of mtDNA mutations is a deficit in energy metabolism and their presence may trigger apoptosis; mtDNA mutations only become physiologically important when a threshold level is exceeded. This level may vary between tissues based on the energy metabolism required for function.

Other Mechanisms of Mitochondrial Damage are Related to Lipid Oxidation and Protein Oxidation

In metabolically active tissues fatty acids are prone to so-called oxidative damage. In addition to producing energy, mitochondria are also a major source of reactive oxygen species, which can lead to lipid peroxidation. In particular, the mitochondrial matrix, which contains DNA, RNA, and numerous enzymes necessary for substrate oxidation, is sensitive to peroxide-induced oxidative damage and needs to be protected against the formation and accumulation of lipids and lipid peroxides. Recent evidence reports that mitochondrial uncoupling is involved in the protection of the mitochondrial matrix against lipid-induced mitochondrial damage. Disturbances in this protection mechanism can contribute to the development of apoptosis.

Ca(2+) mobilization contributes to the more rapid onset of mitochondrial damage, while oxidative damage and lipid peroxidation are involved in the Ca(2+)-independent later onset of mitochondrial damage.

Excess of glutamate can damage the cells because glutamate enhances the permeability to calcium through NMDA receptors located on these neurons. Enhancement of intracellular calcium can induce cell degeneration.

Discussion

Mitochondrial dysfunction plays a role in the pathogenesis of presbycusis, and bioenergetics agents such as creatine, coenzyme Q10, or nicotinamide may be neuroprotective in presbycusis. Coenzyme Q10 inhibits lipid peroxidation by either scavenging free radicals directly or by reducing a-tocopheroxyl radical to a-tocopherol. Coenzyme Q10 protects membrane proteins against oxidation. Coenzyme Q10 also inhibits DNA oxidation in rat liver mitochondria and inhibits DNA strand breaks in human lymphocytes. In the cochlea, coenzyme Q10 presumably prevents lipid oxidation, protein oxidation, and DNA damage [33,34].

Apoptosis can be initiated through two major pathways: the extrinsic or membrane death receptor-dependent pathway and the intrinsic or mitochondrial pathway [35]. The mitochondrial respiratory chain is a powerful source of reactive oxygen species (ROS) and oxidative stress triggers the opening of the mitochondrial permeability transition pores (PTP), that causes the collapse of inner mitochondrial membrane potential and release of pro-apoptotic factors such as cytochrome c a nd/or apoptosis inducing factor (AIF) [36].

Cytochrome c oxidase subunit 3 (COX 3), an essential component in cellular energy metabolism, is encoded in the major arc of the mtDNA genome, is diminished in cells from individuals with presbycusis. This unit is a component of the COX complex: the COX complex is located in the inner mitochondrial membrane and is the last component of the respiratory electron transport chain, which generates the transmembrane electrochemical gradient essential for the production of ATP. This enzyme complex consists of 13 subunits, 10 of which are encoded by nuclear DNA and the remaining 3 are encoded by mtDNA [37].

The deficit of cytochrome c oxidase subunit 3, causes release of cytochrome c and triggers activation of caspase 3, one of the most potent effector's protease, whose activation involves the upstream caspase initiators, caspases 8 and 9, that represent two different signaling pathways in the apoptotic cascade [34].

Ubiquinone 50 or Coenzyme Q10, (CoQ10) is a mobile electron carrier in the mitochondrial electron transfer chain (ETC) that is the major source of ATP in the mitochondria. It participates in the ETC by carrying electrons from complex I (succinate–ubiquinone oxidoreductase) to complex III (ubiquinone–cytochrome c oxidoreductase). Within mitochondria, ubiquinone is reduced by the respiratory chain to its active ubiquinol form, which is an effective antioxidant that prevents lipid peroxidation and mitochondrial damage. In blocking oxidative damage, the ubiquinol is then oxidized to ubiquinone which is reduced back to the active ubiquinol antioxidant by the respiratory chain [34].

Conclusion

In conclusion, the findings illustrated in this chapter represent the experimental basis for the development of a new therapies in the treatment of presbycusis, addressed to prevent lipid peroxidation and mitochondrial damage.

References

[1]   Syka, J. (2002). Plastic changes in the central auditory system after hearing loss, restoration of function, and during learning. *Physiol Rev, 82*, 601-36.

[2]   Markaryan, A.; Nelson, E.G.; Hinojosa, R. (2009). Quantification of the mitochondrial DNA common deletion in presbycusis. *Laryngoscope, 119,* 1184-9.

[3]   Rüttiger, L.; Panford-Walsh, R.; Schimmang, T.; Tan, J.; Zimmermann, U.; Rohbock, K.; Köpschall, I.; Limberger, A.; Müller, M.; Fraenzer, J.T., Cimerman, J.; Knipper, M.(2007). BDNF mRNA expression and protein localization are changed in age-related hearing loss. *Neurobiol Aging, 28*, 586-601.

[4]   Cooper Jr, W.A.; Coleman, J.R.; Newton E.H. (1990). Auditory brainstem responses to tonal stimuli in young and aging rats. *Hear Res , 43*, 171–9.

[5]   Helfert, R.H.; Sommer, T.J.; Meeks, J.; Hofstetter, P.; Hughes, L.F. (1999). Age-related synaptic changes in the central nucleus of the inferior colliculus of Fischer-344 rats. *J Comp Neurol, 406, 285–98.

[6]   Tun, P.A.; McCoy, S.; Wingfield, A. (2009). Aging, hearing acuity, and the attentional costs of effortful listening. *Psychol Aging, 24,* 761-6.

[7]   Gerard, M.; Deleersnijder, A.; Daniëls, V.; Schreurs, S.; Munck, S.; Reumers, V.; Pottel, H.; Engelborghs, Y.; Van den Haute, C.; Taymans, J.M.; Debyser, Z.; Baekelandt, V. (2010). Inhibition of FK506 binding proteins reduces alpha-synuclein aggregation and Parkinson's disease-like pathology. *J Neurosci, 30*, 2454-63.

[8]   Keithley, E.M. & Croskrey, K.L. (1990). Spiral ganglion cell endings in the cochlear nucleus of young and old rats. Hear Res, 49, 169–77.

[9]   Walton, J.P.; Frisina, R.D.; Ison, J.R.; O'Neill, W.E. (1997). Neural correlates of behavioral gap detection in the inferior colliculus of the young CBA mouse. *J Comp Physiol, 181*, 161–76.

[10] Raza, A.; Milbrandt, J.C.; Arneric, S.P.; Caspary, D.M. (1994). Age-related changes in brainstem auditory neurotransmitters: measures of GABA and acetylcholine function. *Hear Res, 77,* 221–30.

[11] Schmiedt, R.A.; Mills, J.H.; Boettcher, F.A. (1996). Age-related loss of activity of auditory-nerve fibres. *J Neurophysiol, 76*, 2799–803.

[12] Taberner, A.M. & Liberman, M.C. (2005). Response properties of single auditory nerve fibres in the mouse. *J Neurophysiol, 93*, 57–69.

[13] Rutherford, L.C.; Nelson, S.B.; Turrigiano, G.G. (1998). BDNF has opposite effects on the quantal amplitude of pyramidal neuron and interneuron excitatory synapses. *Neuron, 21*, 521–30.

[14] Wang, Y. & Manis, P.B. (2005). Synaptic transmission at the cochlear nucleus endbulb synapse during age-related hearing loss in mice. *J Neurophysiol, 94*, 1814–24.

[15] Hamann, I.; Gleich, O.; Klump, G.M.; Kittel, M.C.; Strutz, J. (2004). Age-dependent changes of gap detection in the Mongolian gerbil (Meriones unguiculatus). *J Assoc Res Otolaryngol, 5*, 49–57.

[16]   Knipper, M.; Zinn, C.; Maier, H.; Praetorius, M.; Rohbock, K.; Kopschall, I.; Zimmermann, U. (2000). Thyroid hormone deficiency before the onset of hearing causes irreversible damage to peripheral and central auditory systems. *J Neurophysiol, 83*, 3101–12.

[17]   Ylikoski, J.; Pirvola, U.; Moshnyakov, M.; Palgi, J.; Aruma¨e, U.; Saarma, M. (1993). Expression patterns of neurotrophins and their receptor mRNAs in the rat inner ear. *Hear Res, 65,* 69-78.

[18]   Song, B.N; Li, Y.X.; Han, B.M. (2009). Delayed electrical stimulation and BDNF application following induced deafness in rats. *Acta Oto-Laryngologica*, 129, 142-154.

[19]   Gillespie, L.N.; Clark, G.M.; Bartlett, P.F.; Marzella, P.L. (2003). BDNF induced survival of auditory neurons in vivo: cessation of treatment leads to accelerated loss of survival effects. *J Neurosci Res, 71,* 785-90.

[20]   Hegarty, J.L.; Kay, A.R.; Green, S.H. (1997). Trophic support of cultured spiral ganglion neurons by depolarization exceeds and is additive with that by neurotrophins or cAMP and requires elevation of $[Ca^{2+}]i$ within a set range. *J Neurosci, 17*, 1959-70.

[21]   Autere, A.M.; Lamsa, K.; Kaila, K.; Taira, T. (1999). Synaptic activation of GABAA receptors induces neuronal uptake of Ca^{2+} in adult rat hippocampal slices. *J Neurophysiol, 81*, 811–816.

[22]   Pisani, A.; Calabresi, P.; Centonze, D.; Bernardi, G. (1997). Enhancement of NMDA responses by group I metabotropic glutamate receptor activation in striatal neurones. *Br J Pharmacol, 120,* 1007–1014.

[23]   Sun, W. & Salvi, R.J. (2009). Brain derived neurotrophic factor and neurotrophic factor 3 modulate neurotrasmitter receptor expression on developing spiral ganglion neurons. *Neuroscience, 164*, 1854–1866.

[24]   Acheson, A; Conover, J.C.; Fandl, J.P.; DeChiara, T.M.; Russell, M.; Thadani, A.; Squinto, S.P.; Yancopoulos, G.D.; Lindsay, R.M. (1995). A BDNF autocrine loop in adult sensory neurons prevents cell death. *Nature, 30*, 374, 450-3.

[25]   Hossain, W.A.; D'sa, C.; Morest, D.K. (2006). Site-specific interactions of neurotrophin-3 and fibroblast growth factor (FGF2) in the embryonic development of the mouse cochlear nucleus. *J Neurobiol, 66*, 897–915.

[26]   Feng, J.; Bendiske, J.; Morest, D.K. (2010). Postnatal development of NT3 and TrkC in mouse ventral cochlear nucleus. *J Neurosci Res, 88*, 86-94.

[27]   Berridge, M.V. & Tan, A.S. (1993). Characterization of the cellular reduction of 3-(4,5-dimethylthiazol-2-yl)-2,5-diphenyltetrazolium bromide (MTT): subcellular localization, substrate dependence, and involvement of

mitochondrial electron transport in MTT reduction. *Arch Biochem Biophys 303,* 474–82.

[28] Rossignol, R.; Faustin, B.; Rocher, C.; Malgat, M.; Mazat, J.P.; Letellier, T. (2003). Mitochondrial threshold effects. *Biochem J,* 370, 751–762.

[29] Nelson, E.G. & Hinojosa, R. (2006). Presbycusis: a human temporal bone study of individuals with downward sloping audiometric patterns of hearing loss and review of the literature. *Laryngoscope, 116,* 1–12.

[30] Ueda, N.; Oshima, T.; Ikeda, K.; Abe, K.; Aoki, M.; Takasaka, T. (1998). Mitochondrial DNA deletion is a predisposing cause for sensorineural hearing loss. *Laryngoscope, 108,* 580–584.

[31] Krishnan, K.J.; Greaves, L.C.; Reeve, A.K.; Turnbull, D. (2007). The ageing mitochondrial genome. *Nucleic Acids Res, 35,* 7399–7405.

[32] Fischel-Ghodsian, N.; Kopke, R.D.; Ge, X. (2004). Mitochondrial dysfunction in hearing loss. *Mitochondrion, 4,* 75–694.

[33] Forsmark-Andree, P.; Dallne, G.; Ernster L. (1995). Endogenous ubiquinol prevents protein modification accompanying lipid peroxidation in beef heart submitochondrial particles. *Free Radic Biol Med, 19,* 749-57.

[34] Fetoni, A.R.; Piacentini, R.; Fiorita, A.; Paludetti, G.; Troiani, D. (2009). Water-soluble Coenzyme Q10 formulation (Q-ter) promotes outer hair cell survival in a guinea pig model of noise induced hearing loss (NIHL). *Brain Res, 1257,* 108–16.

[35] Van De Water, T.R., Lallemend, F., Eshraghi, A.A., Ahsan, S., He, J., Guzman, J., Polak, M., Malgrange, B., Lefebvre, P.P., Staecker, H., Balkany, T.J. (2004). Caspases, the enemy within, and their role in oxidative stress-induced apoptosis of inner ear sensory cells. *Otol. Neurol, 25,* 627–632.

[36] Reed, J.C. (2000). Mechanisms of apoptosis. *Am. J. Pathol, 157,* 1415–1430.

[37] Johnson, M.A.; Turnbull, D.M.; Dick, D.J.; Sherratt, H.S.A. (1983). A partial deficiency of cytochrome c oxidase in chronic progressive external ophthalmoplegia. *J Neurol Sci,* 60, 31–53.

In: Neuroplasticity in the Auditory Brainstem   ISBN 978-1-61761-949-6
Editor: Angelo Salami, pp. 45-62   © 2011 Nova Science Publishers, Inc.

Chapter IV

Neuroplasticity in the Auditory System after Hearing Loss

Pablo Gil-Loyzaga

Professor of Neurobiology of Hearing. Director of the Department of
Ophthalmology and Oto-Rhyno-Laryngology, Faculty of Medicine,
University Complutense of Madrid, Spain

Abstract

Neuroplasticity is the ability of neurons to adapt their connection tree's
configuration and shape to their functional requirements. This capacity is
especially relevant as the morpho-functional base to processes essential to
individual's survival, such as learning and memory. Thus, neurons can
modify their own function by using short or long-term potentiation or
depression as an expression of current activity. Also, neuroplasticity is linked
to neurons and neuronal circuitry recovery after damage or lesion, as well as
to the acquisition and maintenance of language, the most differential activity
of human beings. Neuroplasticity is required to organize and stabilize
language circuitry during human maturation, but it is also clearly involved in
the acquisition of a second, third and subsequent languages. A deep
permanent hearing loss is usually related to an important cochlear lesion (f. i.
acoustic trauma, hair cell and / or neuron degeneration) or auditory nerve
damage where afferent auditory nerve terminals on cochlear nuclei neurons

could be highly altered. Cochlea removal has been used to analyze brainstem cochlear nuclei neuroplasticity. In this experimental model the early disappearance of big primary afferent buttons projecting on cochlear nuclei neurons was noticed. These big buttons dramatically disappeared leaving large areas of neuron membrane surface devoid of synaptic contacts. Later, round small buttons, GAP-43 positive, covered these areas. It seems evident that these didn't correspond to previously removed primary afferents, but to other neuron types: projections to other auditory pathway structures on cochlear nuclei (f. i. olivary complex, etc.) or internal connection from other neurons at the cochlear nucleus. This finding clearly indicates that adult neurons keep enough ability to reorganize auditory circuits after lesion, but this new reorganization could not correspond to the previous circuitry.

Keywords*:* neuroplasticity, regeneration, brainstem cochlear nuclei complex, auditory pathway

Introduction

Neuroplasticity has been defined as the ability of neurons to adapt their circuitry of connections to any relevant change of their activity. Although neuroplasticity is a simple concept, it is largely used in the nervous system. Many processes such as neural development, maturity, or those occurring after injury or during memory or learning, amongst others, are dependent on neuroplasticity.

Classical studies on the nervous tissue let scientists to conclude that, with exception of development or regeneration after damage, neurons and circuitry were only involved in sending neural messages. Some time ago, a generally accepted hypothesis suggested that mature/adult nervous system remained "*quiescent*" from a structural point of view, even though there could be the more active/functional tissue in the body. This hypothesis was insufficient to explain a large number of situations that were progressively analyzed, in particular learning and memory. If neural circuitry was "*definitively fixed*" during development and maturation, the possibility to establish any kind of permanent conditioned behavior in adult animals should be excluded. This hypothesis was found to be progressively in clear contrast with findings obtained from experimental models. It was evident that a persistent activity increase in a chemical synapse linked to stimulation resulted, firstly in an increase of functional capacity and later in the reorganization of the synaptic tree. It is now well accepted that central and peripheral nervous system are the result of a long and complex remodelling plastic process. But also, neural recovery after any damage or chronic sensory deprivation could be hard to explain without neuroplasticity processes [1-7]. An increasing number of experiments concluded that nerve regeneration and neuroplasticity, largely identified during development, are still present in the adulthood [5].

Neuroplasticity, in the auditory cortex, has been involved in learning tasks [8] being the main neural mechanism leading to animal survival, by using complementary psycho-physiological processes, such as learning and memory. Animal survival depends on the ability of the nervous system to integrate external and internal information. All this information, obtained throughout specialized sensory receptors, must be analyzed and integrated in cross-modal interactions [1, 2]. But, it will only be useful if new information might be compared to previous experience and if it could be incorporated using memory tasks. Therefore, sensory cross-modal interactions and neuroplasticity become absolutely necessary for adaptation to new environmental situations and animal's survival [2, 4].

Sensory systems are much less independent that it was classically considered. First of all, sensory information must be integrated in the brain cortex to reach an useful meaning. This has been largely shown by magneto-encephalography studies, when the brain activity was tracked during 600 ms after sensory stimulation. In fact, cortical activity exhibits a sequential pattern that could be related to the learning process. Sensory stimulation patterns reaching the corresponding cortical area, after filtering by the successive nuclei of the pathway, need to establish some interrelationship [cross modal interactions] with other sensory patterns, that were concomitantly learnt in other brain areas. Thus, the cross-modal interactions are absolutely necessary for the correct brain integration of sensory information but, in particular, to prepare the adequate response [9, 10]. Up to now, it is accepted that cross-modal interaction is the most common brain function for management of sensory information [9]. It is clear from experimental models of sensory deprivation [f. i. blindness, deafness, etc.] [10] and their corresponding clinics.

But cross-modal interactions need that neurons and neural circuits remain with the enough plastic ability to reorganize their connections, in particular when neural activity increases/decreases, during new tasks, learning, etc. All neurons, from both central and peripheral nervous system, are able of a plastic response after chemical factors stimulation, even when these cells are developed in culture conditions [12,13]. The search of factors involved in the organization or reorganization of neural circuits and in the guidance of nerve fibers, toward their specific targets, is highly relevant to understand neuroplasticity. Experimental research, both in vitro and in conventional animal models (typically rodents), could provide enough information for a potential therapeutic use of the substances involved in such processes. The search of substances, but also the patterns of use, has become highly relevant and requires a separate comment.

Molecular Mechanisms of Neuroplasticity

A great number of substances are required to stimulate neurons during neuroplasticity processes. The more relevant events of neuroplasticity take place during nervous system development [13] using a "cascade" pattern: each substance acts before and after another, in an ordered and consecutive line. But also re-growing nerve fibers, after damage, are submitted to the same substances and use the same pattern of action [see reviews for auditory neurons in: 1, 4, 13]. Some chemical agents stimulate neuroplasticity from the distance, while others act from the vicinity of the target (neuron affected). These substances were firstly identified by Levi Montalcini and are currently called as neurotrophic factors [14].

Some substances create "an adequate environment", as it is the case of neurotrophic factors, acting on the whole neuronal sprouting but also helping neuron survival [12,14]. All neurons are submitted to the action of neurotrophic factors, hormones or other substances, including neurotransmitters. In fact, the collaborative action of several trophic factors (bFGF, NGF, EGF, TGFa, GDNF, NT-3 and BDNF or other) [12,14-16] and hormones (insulin or IGF-1) serve to maintain or protect neurons and stimulate general fasciculation and neuroplasticity [17] (Table 1). Neurotrophic factors act throughout cell-membrane tyrosine-kinase receptors (TrkA, TrkB or TrkC) [15,16,18,19], that are genetically coded in any kind of neuron in a specific and particular manner (Table 1).

But the organization of the highly complex neural circuits, as in the case of the adult auditory pathway, requires also guidance of elements serving to correctly address nerve fibers to their corresponding targets. The specific "pathways of guidance" have been analyzed in many parts of central and peripheral nervous system, being the developing neural crest a paradigm. It seems evident that neurons are guided by using extracellular matrix proteins (laminin and others), cell-adhesion molecules (NCAM, NgCAM, LCAM, cadherins), etc. [see reviews in 1,4,12,20] (Table 1).

Other substances could also have the ability to specifically attract nerve sprouting to very restricted and defined targets. Only this possibility might serve to the organization of highly precise and complex circuits, as it occurs in the central nervous system. It can be generally considered that target cells, well defined and highly precise elements, could attract some particular fibers from their corresponding "partner", inside of specific neural circuits.

Table 1.

Neurotrophic factors	
Stimulatory Factors	**Inhibitory NT Factors**
Laminin	Myelin inhibitory protein
Fibronectin	Axonal inhibitory molecules
Collagen	Tenascin
N-cadheryns	Neurotransmitters
NCAM (NgCAM, LCAM)	Semaphorins & Netrins
Neurofascin, Retinoic acid	
Neurotransmitters	
Semaphorins & Netrins	

The existence of some substances involved in such a process was suggested largely before their identification. In fact, at the beginning of the 20th century Ramón y Cajal [21] suggested the existence of some factors acting during neural development. From its own words he suggested the presence during development of some *"chemical substance for nerve fibre attraction"*, this substance serves to *"nerve growth cones to recognize, and directionally respond to increasing gradients of diffusible substances released by their targets"* [21].

These agents let nerve fibers grow and precisely reach their corresponding targets [21]. They could be probably complementary to the action of neurotrophic factors. It was promptly suggested that such substances should be released by the targets. They might generate a "concentration gradient" in their very close neighboring that serve to the wandering fibers as a *"safety path in a forest"*. Some substances such as neurotransmitters, or other neuroactive substances, ions and hormones, were involved. Neuroactive substances or neurotransmitters, directly released even from immature neurons or sensory cells, could clearly guide growing nerve fibers until reaching the target [12,20]. The same mechanism could be *"re-install"* after nerve injury and degeneration.

Nowadays, apart from classical neurotrophic factors, only some other few substances have been identified as potential agents of these processes. Neurotransmitters such as glutamate [acting on the NMDA receptor] and GABA seem to be stimulating agents of neuroplasticity (Table I), at least on neurons cultured in vitro. Some authors have indicated that NMDA receptor and glutamate could be considered as the *"neural circuit sculptors"* [7,22], being specially relevant the role of the NMDA-glutamate system in memory tasks. Hence, both glutamate and GABA might be relevant substances eliciting neuroplasticity [2,7,23]. A repeated glutamate release, which acts on the postsynaptic membrane throughout ionotropic and/or metabotropic receptors [24], eases the influx of Ca^{2+}, which is a potent neuroplasticity agent [15,25]. Glutamate might stimulate the quick axon or dendrite filopodia neurofasciculation [26]. In-vitro experiments added relevant information. When glutamate or GABA were administered in-vitro to isolated spiral ganglion neurons, it clearly elicited neuron fasciculation and organization of *"simple circuits"*, that were absent in control experiments [3,7,13]. These studies need to be re-analyzed using degeneration-regeneration in-vivo models, involving not only developing but also adult animals. However, it seems evident that the sprouting or neurofasciculation obtained in-vivo models will be the result of the complementary action of many substances acting in a cascade sequence.

Neuroplasticity and Auditory System

Hearing must be considered one of the most critical systems involved in animal survival, protecting it against both depredators and physical natural agents and phenomena. This is due to the fact that sound information can stimulate auditory receptor (and then pathway) from a very long distance, allowing any kind of early and quick response. In contrast, other sensory systems need very particular environmental conditions (light and adequate proximity for vision) or directly the close contact between the stimulus and the receptor (taste, smell, pain, etc.). The particular relevance that exhibits the auditory system becomes very special for humans, making hearing probably the most important sensory system for humans. In fact, hearing and fine analysis of complex sound and messages allowed developing oral language, an exclusive characteristic of human species [27].

Hearing is linked to the sound learning [words] and language comprehension, thus it becomes much more psycho-physiologically relevant for humans than for other species, including big apes. The relevant position of the auditory system in the whole functional activity of the human brain can be evidenced from the development of the oral language in the human species (see comments below), but also by many other examples. Several psycho-pathologies might be more related with the auditory system than expected. Some examples might be: epileptic attacks elicited by particular sounds, voices perceived *"in the brain or head"* as a relevant aspect for schizophrenic crisis, or the relationship between hearing and brain degenerative diseases. As a good example for this last group, Alzheimer's disease can be mentioned. This progressive, degenerative and irreversible brain disorder results in intellectual impairment, disorientation and dementia. But, some of the best psychotherapies to slow down the progression of this disease are based in musical therapy, exercises which include remembering list of words, etc.

At the physiological level, hearing can be defined as the organization centre of the cross-modal interactions. For instance, each word heard first reaches the auditory cortex and then immediately elicits high defined patterns of activity in the rest of the cortical areas. Cross-modal interactions allow access to the whole information - *"the concept"*- contained in a specific word. The brain path for this function is mediated by commissural nerve fibers; both inter-hemispheric (between areas of brain hemispheres) and intra-hemispheric (all functional areas) connections are involved. In that cases, the cortical circuit supporting the actual and complete comprehension of a word starts at the auditory primary area, where frequencies [tonotopic area] but also complex patterns (secondary area) are analyzed [28]. From the auditory cortex the functional activity reaches other cortical areas [visual cortex, olfactory cortex, somato-sensory cortex, hippocampus, etc]. For normal hearing people, this interaction, carried out in the first 600 ms after stimulation, is required to really understand the concept linked to a word. Of course, in the case of absence or not correct function of auditory inputs, neuroplasticity enables other sensory systems [vision, etc.] to occupy this leadership function with more or less accuracy. Sensory processing, specially relevant for hearing, is carried out by highly complex neural circuits that are not static or immutable at all [10,17].

Other particular characteristic of the hearing-speech system in human species is the long time needed for learning of a language. The acquisition of an enough knowledge of a particular language, to be enough useful for individual social interaction, varies with: 1) each language, 2) the previous background and 3) the age or maturation of the individual. The learning of the first language (also called *"the maternal language"*) is relatively long. In normal environment and social conditions, involves until the five-six years. It is due that language learning is coincident with the whole maturation and acquisition of many other attitudes and social roles. However, the learning of the maternal language, clearly based in circuits of sensory cross-modal interactions, is so deep in terms of neural circuit development, that definitively establish *"a priority neural pathway"* that remains for the rest of the life. This has been clearly observed by using highly sensitive methods of cortical activity (f. i. magnetoencephalography) when bilingual subjects were explored. In fact, the acquisition of the also called *"foreign languages"* (that could be better called the second, third, etc. languages) requires a very active neuroplasticity.

A deep learning of *"foreign languages"*, to reach the actual bilingual status, requires a complex reorganization of the cross-modal interactions. This is only possible in young people or in previously trained ones (f. i. people spoken several languages, musicians or so). This is because each concept usually has a different word (with its corresponding phonetic pattern) for each language. However, the primary analysis of the auditory pathway is based in the frequency analysis of each sound (which is particularly relevant for complex sounds). A new phonetic pattern will stimulate a different region of the auditory primary cortex than in the precedent (f.i. maternal) language. The main problem during language learning will be neuroplasticity required by the association of each specific auditory cortex areas to other sensory cortex by using *"concepts"* and avoiding the primary stimulation (frequencies). Even though that learning and memory in the auditory pathway remain very active long lifespan it will be only really possible in young or specially trained subjects.

Neuroplasticity processes are required during language learning and its maturation, but also during the acquisition of a second, third. etc. language, Neuroplasticity is also highly relevant for music learning and recognition and in related memory tasks. This very fine process, conducted by a large number of substances and conditions acting in an ordered cascade sequence, can also result in failed neuroplasticity situations. If the system NMDA-glutamate has been considered at the molecular level as the neural circuit sculptor, it must be defined that for human brain organization *"the language"* might be the truthful *"sculptor of the human brain"* [22,28].

Hearing and neuroplasticity are closely related not only to speech or music learning and memory but also during the regeneration processes. Neuroplasticity linked to recovery after lesion or damage might be useful, but also might generate negative or inadequate functional results. Hence, an abnormal neuroplasticity might derive in malformation syndromes during development or maturation. Also, an inadequate connectivity after nerve or synaptic regeneration (elicited by noise trauma etc.) might derive in chronic auditory alterations [29-30], such as deafness or tinnitus [29-32].

The adequate stimulation of neuroplasticity could be useful for inner ear or auditory pathway therapy. By using appropriate drugs or substances, it could provide a complementary enhancement to cochlear implants. The extensive use of cochlear implants has proven to be a very useful tool for hearing recovering of deep deaf people [12]. But, there has been identified some particular deficiencies for cochlear implants that make it hard to correctly hear music or establish subtle differences among voices and tones, amongst others. It has been suggested that stimulation of cochlear ganglion neuroplasticity might be certainly useful to improve cochlear implant accuracy. The combined use of cochlear implantation and neurotrophic substances could serve for two main purposes: the delay or blocking of neuron degeneration linked to atrophy by loss of activity during deafness and the achievement of better interactions between neurons and the implant.

Some relevant questions remain completely opened when the combination of cochlear implants technology and trophic factors administration, or any other neuroplasticity stimulation, are planned. First of all, the selection of the appropriate substances to be delivered throughout the implant remains controversial. Also, a not minor or avoidable question will be the selection of the appropriate timing and sequence of treatment with the chosen substances [12]. A very relevant message to be delivered to clinicians is the *"the miracle substance doesn't exist"*; in fact, probably the final solution will be the selection of a combination of several drugs acting together on unlike targets. The use of micropumps for continuous, or sporadic, perfusion could also serve as useful paths for trophic substances. It seems clear that the research of auditory nerve neuroplasticity opens unexpected perspectives for the deafness therapy in the forthcoming future. All these comments make very attractive neuroplasticity studies for both ENT specialists and basic research scientists.

Neurons, Growth Cones and Neuroplasticity

The whole circuitry that constitutes the organization of the nervous system (including sensory receptor systems and pathways) is basically built during embryo development. This basic pattern is genetically-determined and is dependent of the species considered. However, it includes some *"very small"* individual variations that are also genetically determined but also epigenetically dependent of embryo environment, in particular of the maternal-fetal relationship. This includes temperature, homeostasis (ions, etc.), hormones, vitamins, essential amino acids and other nutritional components that might influence on the nervous system at birth. A classical example of such influences is the relevance of thyroid hormone on the maturation of the auditory receptor [see comments in 33]. Therefore, from the beginning of the independent life on the progressive adding of individual experience (f.i. learning, memory process etc.) actively contributes to the complexity and maturation of these basic neural patterns [17,34].

The neuron elongations that let growth to a dendrite or an axon, during development / maturation or after neural damage, have been classically called as *"growth cones"* [35]. These growth cones are high complex cytoplasm cytopodes that establish neuron contacts and initiate synaptogenesis [36,37]. Growth cones exhibit a highly motile behavior [35] in response to specific activation, generally linked to the presence of neurotrophic factors, that modulate (positively or negatively) the directional growth of these structures. Positive attractants are semaphorins, ephrins, netrins etc.. All of these stimulate neurite growing towards a specific target by two complementary actions: the reorganization of the neuron cytoskeleton and the progressive addition of new cell membrane [12]. This neuroplasticity process lets during animal development the organization of neural circuits reaching their final modeling by the stimulation/inhibition induced by chemical factors. Neurites, from developing and adult animals, can add new membrane. It has been established in experimental models that neurite exhibited multiple and widely regions where membrane can be added [38]. Therefore after lesion or damage adult nerve fibers still can be recovered by such a process [38]. The study of genetic and epigenetic factors involved in neuroplasticity is, probably, one of the main challenges for the forthcoming inner ear research.

Neuroplasticity and Experimental Deafness by Cochlear Induced Lesion

The analysis of the effects of deafness and subsequent neuroplasticity on auditory nerve pathway, from brainstem on, is not a simple matter at all. This is due to the neuroplasticity process itself. If the peripheral lesion of the auditory receptor involves only a limited number of neurons, the high capacity of neuroplasticity process could cover the synapses lost at the brainstem, with minor morphological effects difficult to explore. However, the auditory function of such a *"recovered pathway"* might be physiologically not good enough. This clearly indicates that in order to explore the neuroplasticity process, the experimental models chosen need to include a more dramatic neuron loose. Animal model (rats and others) submitted to experimental cochlea removal or auditory nerve section seems adequate to analyze the complete auditory deprivation and subsequent neuroplasticity in the auditory pathway [6, 10, 11, 39-41].

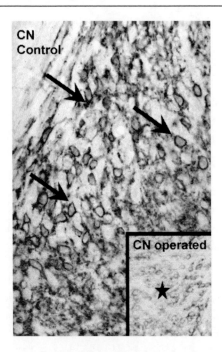

Figure 1. Microscopy photograph of rat cochlear nuclei (CN) 15 days after cochlear removal. Immunostaining to identify Syp (synaptophysin) expression. Arrows indicate CN neurons surrounded by nerve endings containing Syp in a control animal. Detail shows the dramatic reduction of Syp expression (star) in rat cochlear nuclei 15 days after cochlear removal.

The effects of unilateral cochlea removal on auditory pathway have been analyzed after short to long periods after surgery [5,6]. Two interesting neural proteins have been analyzed: synaptophysin (Syp), a calcium-dependent synaptic protein, and growth association protein (GAP-43) present in developing and regenerating nerve-ending buttons. The Syp expression allows to identify different kind of synaptic buttons in the brainstem cochlear nuclei (Figure 1).

Previous publications [5,6] let us recognize at least three main cochlear nuclei degeneration / recovery phases after cochlea removal.

1. First Phase: Acute Cochlear Nuclei Degeneration [5,6]

Early after cochlea removal (one day on) some neural changes were found including: edema images within auditory nerve fiber (the remaining part inside cochlear nuclei), even though neurons of the cochlear nuclei still exhibited a normal shape. Early cochlear nuclei neuron death was found after cochlea removal in some particular susceptible animals [40,42]. A very early reduction of Syp expression was noted in rats [5,6] and in guinea pigs after cochlea removal [43], which remained for a very large period.

2. Second Phase: Stabilization of Lesions and Neuroplasticity

Since a week after cochlear removal a new period, of around 15 days, was characterized by two facts in particular: 1) the increase of neuron cell death was observed and 2) the clear appearance of neuroplasticity. Also a significant change in Syp expression was noted (compare Figure 1 and detail at the same figure). While the ventral cochlear nucleus appeared quite devoid of big end-bulbs of Held, some small buttons containing Syp were still found surrounding neuron cell bodies [5,6]. This indicates the complete loss of primary afferent fibers instead of the healthy immunostained small buttons (Figure 1 detail). Small buttons represent internal connections and fibers coming from other brainstem nuclei (superior olivary complex, etc).

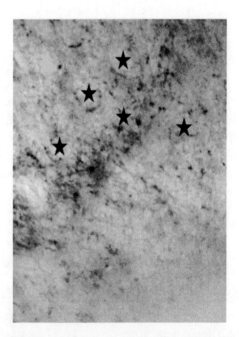

Figure 2. Microscopy photograph of rat cochlear nuclei (CN) 15 days after cochlear removal. Neurons appeared (stars) surrounded by round small nerve endings containing GAP-43 protein.

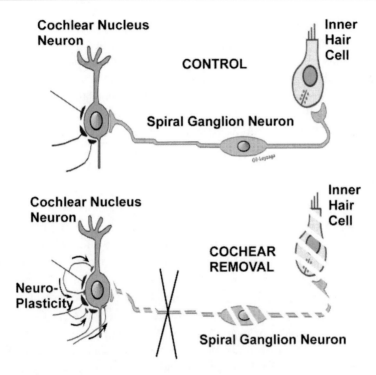

Figure 3. Schematic representation of a cochlear sensory cell (inner hair cell) connected through the spiral ganglion neuron to the cochlear nuclei neurons. Cochlear removal stimulates neuroplasticity around cochlear nuclei neurons.

At this period, some still scarce but evident signs of neuroplasticity were noticed. The expression of growth association protein (GAP-43), a transient neural protein linked to neural development and recovery after lesion (Figure 2), was used as a marker of regenerating axons [44]. Some neurons showed small nerve endings and punctae containing GAP-34 around their somata, indicating the presence of an increasing neuroplasticity processes. These nerve endings might correspond to fibers projecting on the cochlear nuclei from commissural fibers on the other no-deprived side [45] or other auditory pathway nuclei [46,47].

3. Third Phase: Neuroplasticity and CN Reorganization

One month or later after cochlear removal a last phase may be identified. Some cochlear nuclei neurons still degenerate but the most important finding was that at this period the regeneration process is relevant [5,6]. The GAP-43 expression was more intense than in previous periods. Now, neurons also exhibited a relevant number of Syp containing nerve endings around cell bodies. This clearly indicates that the regenerative process inside cochlear nuclei includes the organization of new circuits (Figure 3). These new circuits seemed to be established between projections of other brainstem neurons (contralateral cochlear nuclei, superior olivary complex, descending auditory pathway, etc.) and de-afferented cochlear nuclei neurons after cochlear removal.

Conclusion

Neuroplasticity studies seem to be relevant from the experimental models (including in vitro isolated cells, animal model deprivation etc.) until clinical research. Neuroplasticity could serve to answer many opened questions, hard to answer without considering neuroplasticity processes as intimately linked to any auditory lesion, damage or deprivation. Neuroplasticity is a very complex process that involves many substances that positively or negatively control the organization and recovery of neural circuits. Nevertheless, not all neuroplasticity processes end with a correct functional system and some hearing and speech pathologies might derivate from an abnormal neuroplasticity. Thus, the deep analysis of the factors involved in neuroplasticity could lead to understand the pathogenesis of diseases (f. i. deafness, tinnitus, dyslexia, etc.). In contrast, the correct management of neuroplasticity might have a large number of applications in current and future therapies (f.i. cochlear implants, stem cells and nerve regeneration). Further research must be devoted to evaluate the factors that, alone or combined, are involved in neuroplasticity and the critical periods of administration.

Acknowledgments

This review has been supported by a CCG 07-UCM/SAL-2992 grant to "Cátedra de Neurobiología de la Audición" from the Complutense University of Madrid [Spain]

References

[1]   Gil-Loyzaga P, Neuroplasticidad y Sistema Auditivo. In: Suarez C, Gil-Carcedo LM, Marco J, Medina J, Ortega P, Trinidad J, editors. Tratado Otorrinolaringología & Cirugía Cabeza & Cuello Vol. II. 2nd ed. Panamericana; 2007. p. 1057-67.

[2]   Nitsche MA, Liebetanz D, Paulus W, Tergau F. Pharmacological characterisation and modulation of neuroplasticity in humans. *Curr Neuropharmacol.* 2005;3:217-29.

[3]   Syka J. Plastic changes in the central auditory system after hearing loss, restoration of function, and during learning. *Physiol Rev.* 2002;82:601-36

[4]   Gil-Loyzaga P. Neuroplasticity in the auditory system. *Europ Rev ENT.* 2005;126/4:203-8.

[5]   Gil-Loyzaga P, Iglesias MC, Carricondo F, Bartolome M, Rodríguez F, Poch-Broto J. Cochlear nuclei neuroplasticity after auditory nerve and cochlea removal. *Audiological Medicine* 2009:7/1:29 - 39.

[6]   Gil-Loyzaga P, Carricondo F, Bartolome M,Iglesias MC, Rodríguez F, Poch-Broto J. Cellular and molecular bases of neuroplasticity: brainstem effects after cochlear damage. *Acta Otolaryngol* [Stockh] 2009: 10:1-8

[7]   Haberny KA, Paule MG, Scallet AC, Sistare FD, Lester DS, et al. Ontogeny of the N-Methyl-D-Aspartate [NMDA] Receptor System and Susceptibility to Neurotoxicity. *Toxicol Sci.* 2002;68:9-17.

[8]   Irvine DR. Auditory cortical neuroplasticity: does it provide evidence for cognitive processing in the auditory cortex?. *Her Res.* 2007;229:158-70

[9]   Díaz Arribas MJ, Pardo-Hervás P, Tabares-Lavado M, Rios-Lago M, Maestú F. Plasticidad del sistema nervioso central y estrategias de tratamiento para la reprogramación sensorimotora: comparación de dos casos de accidente cerebrovascular isquémico en el territorio de la arteria cerebral media. *Rev Neurol,* 2006;42153-8.

[10] Shimojo S, Sams L. Sensory modalities are not separate modalities: plasticity and interactions. *Curr Op Neurobiol* 2001;11:505-9.

[11] Gil-Loyzaga P. Neuroplasticity as a useful tool in otology and cochlear implantation. en: *"Surgery of the Ear - Current Topics".* Editor O. Nuri Ozgirgin. Edit. Rekmay Publish. LTD. (Ankara Turquía). pág. 479-483.

[12] Gil-Loyzaga P. Biological bases of neuroplasticity - in vivo and in vitro studies: Interest for the auditory system. *Audiological Medicine* 2009:7/1:2-10.

[13] Gil-Loyzaga P. Neurotransmitters and neuroplasticity during cochlear development: in vivo and in vitro studies. *Audiological Medicine* 2009:7/1:11-21.

[14] Levi-Montalcini R. Developmental neurobiology and the natural history of nerve growth factor. *Ann Rev Neurosci.* 1982;5:341-62.

[15] Barbacid M. Neurotrophic factors and their receptors. *Current Op Cell Biol* 1995;7,148-55.

[16] Korsching S. The neurotrophic factor concept: a reexamination. *J. Neurosci.* 1993;13:2739-48.

[17] Bergado-Rosado JA, Almaguer-Melian W. Cellular mechanisms of neuroplasticity. *Rev Neurol.* 2000;31:1074-95.

[18] Chao MV, Hempstead BL. p75 and Trk: a two-receptor system. *TINS.* 1995;18:321-6.

[19] Pirvola U, Hallböök F, Xing-Qun L, Virkkala J, Saarma M, et al. Expression of neurotrophins and Trk receptors in the developing, adult, and regenerating avian cochlea. *J Neurobiol.* 1997;33:1019-33.

[20] Castro Soubriet F. Moléculas quimiotrópicas como mecanismo de orientación del crecimiento axonal y de la migración neuronal durante el desarrollo del sistema nervioso de los mamíferos. *Rev Neurol.* 2001;33:54-68.

[21] Ramón y Cajal S. Acción neurotrópica de los epitelios [Algunos detalles sobre el mecanismo genético de las ramificaciones nerviosas intra-epiteliales, sensitivas y sensoriales]. *Trab Lab Inv Biol.* 1919;17:81-228.

[22] Gil-Loyzaga P: Fisiología del receptor auditivo. In: P. Gil-Loyzaga. Fisiología y fisiopatología de la cóclea. *Suppl Act ORL. SANED Publ. Madrid.* 2005:1: 1-7.

[23] Emerit MB, Riad M, Hamon M. Trophic effects of neurotransmitters during brain maturation. *Biol Neonate.* 1992;62,4:193-201.

[24] Puel JL, Ruel J, Guitton M, Wang J, Pujol R. The inner hair cell synaptic complex: physiology, pharmacology and new therapeutic strategies. *Audiol Neurootol.* 2002;7:49-54.

[25] Zamanillo D, Sprengel R, Hvalby O, Jensen V, Burnashev N, et al. Importance of AMPA receptors for hippocampal synaptic plasticity but not for spatial learning. *Science* 1999;284:1805-11.

[26] Portera-Cailliau C, Yuste R. On the function of dendritic filopodia. *Rev Neurol.* 2001;33:1158-66.

[27] Deacon TW. Prefrontal cortex and symbol learning: Why a brain capable of language evolved only once. In BM Velichkovsky, DM Rumbaugh.

Communicating meaning: The evolution and development of language. LEA Publ. New York. 1996:103-38.

[28] Gil-Loyzaga P: Estructura y función de la corteza auditiva. Bases de la vía auditiva ascendente. In: E Salesa, E Perelló, A Bonavida. Tratado de Audiologia. Masson-Elsevier Ed. *Barcelona* 2005:23-38.

[29] Moller AR. Symptoms and signs caused by neural plasticity. *Neurol Res.* 2001;23:565-72.

[30] Jin YM, Godfrey DA. Effects of cochlear ablation on muscarinic acetylcholine receptor biding in the rat cochlear nucleus. *J Neurosci Res.* 2006;83:157-66.

[31] Bartels H, Staal MJ, Albers FWJ. Tinnitus and neural plasticity of the brain. *Otol Neurotol* 2007;28:178-84.

[32] Cacace AT. Expanding the biological bases of tinnitus: cross-modal origins and the role of neuroplasticity. *Hear Res.* 2003;175:112-32.

[33] Gil-Loyzaga P: Histochemistry of glycoconjugates of the auditory receptor. *Progress in Histochemistry and Cytochemistry. Gustav Fischer Verlag [Stuttgart-Jena-Lübeck-Ulm]* 1997;32/1:1-78.

[34] Toyama K, Komatsu Y, Yamamoto N, Kurotami T, Yamada K. In vitro approach to visual cortical development and plasticity. *Neurosci Res* 1991;12:57-71.

[35] Letourneau PC. Regulation of nerve fiber elongation suring embryogenesis. In WT Greennough, JM Juraska. *Developmental Neuropsychobiology.* Acad. Press Ibc. Harc. Brace Jovanovich Publish. Oralndo USA. 1986, 2:33-71.

[36] Bufill E, Carbonell E. Are symbolic behaviour and neuroplasticity an example of gene-culture coevolution? *Rev Neurol* 2004:39:48-55.

[37] Jones TA, Kleim JA, Greenough WT. Synaptogenesis and dendritic growth in the cortex opposite unilateral sensorymotor cortex damage in adult rats: a quantitative electron microscopic examination. *Brain Res* 1996;773:142-8.

[38] Futerman AH, Banker GA. The economics of neurite outgrowth. The addition of new membrane to growing axons. *Trends Neurosci.* 1996;19:144-9.

[39] Illing RB, Reisch A. Specific plasticity responses to unilaterally decreased or increased hearing intensity in the adult cochlear nucleus and beyond. *Hearing Res.* 2006; 216, 189-97.

[40] Rubel EW, Hyson RL, Durham D. Afferent regulation of neurons in the brain stem auditory system. *J. Neurobiol.* 1990;21:169-96.

[41] Kraus KS, Illing RB. Cell death or survival: molecular and connectional
      conditions for olivocochlear neurons after axotomy. *Neuroscience*
      2005;134:467- 81.

[42] *Mostafapour* SP, Cochran SL, del Puerto NM, Rubel EW. Patterns of cell
      death in mouse anteroventral cochlear nucleus neurons after unilateral
      cochlea removal. *J Comp Neurol* 2000:426:561-71.

[43] Benson CG, Gross JS, Suneja SK, Potashner SJ. Synaptophysin
      immunoreactivity in the cochlear nucleus after unilateral cochlear or
      ossicular removal. *Synapse* 1997;25:243-57.

[44] Verhhagen J, Van Hooff COM, Edwards PM, De Graan PNE, Oestreicher
      AB, Schotman P et al. The kinase C substrate protein B-50 and axonal
      regeneration. *Brain Res Bull* 1986;17:737-41.

[45] Shore SE, Godfrey DA, Helfert RH, Altschuler RA, Bledsoe SC Jr.
      Connections between the cochlear nuclei in guinea pig. *Hear Res.*
      1992;62:16-26.

[46] Ryan AF, Keithley EM, Wang ZX, Schwartz IR. Collaterals from lateral
      and medial olivocochlear efferent neurons innervate different regions of the
      cochlear nucleus and adjacent brainstem. *J Comp Neurol.* 1990;300:572-82.

[47] Shore SE, Helfert RH, Bledsoe SC Jr, Altschuler RA, Godfrey DA.
      Descending projections to the dorsal and ventral divisions of the cochlear
      nucleus in guinea pig. *Hear Res.* 1991;52:255-68.

In: Neuroplasticity in the Auditory Brainstem   ISBN 978-1-61761-949-6
Editor: Angelo Salami, pp. 63-73   © 2011 Nova Science Publishers, Inc.

Chapter V

Hearing Loss and Balance Dysfunction in Children

Michael S. Cohen and Margaretha L. Casselbrant
Division of Pediatric Otolaryngology. University of Pittsburgh School of
Medicine, Pittsburgh, PA, USA

Introduction

An expanding body of literature continues to demonstrate that hearing loss is frequently associated with vestibular dysfunction, balance disturbances, and delays in motor development. Hearing loss, typically classified as either conductive or sensorineural, is the most common sensory loss in humans. 1 to 3 out of every 1000 children born in the United States have permanent hearing loss.[1] While the most obvious impact of hearing loss is its effect on communication, disturbances in balance, posture, gait, learning, and reading acuity are increasingly recognized. Early detection of functional deficits in the hearing impaired child may enable early intervention and improve functional outcomes in this important group.

This chapter will summarize the existing literature relating to balance and vestibular dysfunction in children with hearing loss. The developmental impact of these conditions will be examined and the role of early intervention will be explored.

Sensorineural Hearing Loss

1. Balance and Vestibular Dysfunction in SHNL

In light of the close anatomic and phylogenetic relationship between the cochlea and the vestibule, it is no surprise that vestibular dysfunction in patients with profound SNHL has been observed. Furthermore, the prevalence of vestibular dysfunction has been shown to correlate with severity of hearing loss. [Arnvig 1955, Sandberg 1965] Postural control, locomotion, and gait are often impaired in children with profound SNHL and bilateral vestibular hypofunction.

In the adult literature, vestibular hypofunction has been demonstrated in anywhere from 25-100% of patients with severe to profound bilateral SNHL. For example, Krause and colleagues assessed 47 subjects aged 16-83 years with bilateral severe-profound SNHL for vertigo symptoms and vestibular function prior to cochlear implantation. 53% reported balance problems; 40% had abnormal rotational chair testing and 60% had abnormal bithermal caloric testing. [Krause 2008] In a second study by the same group, 65% of adult CI candidates had abnormal vestibular evoked myogenic potential (VEMP) measurements preoperatively, indicating saccular dysfunction. [Krause 2009] Ribari and colleagues studied 24 children and 42 adults with bilateral severe-profound SNHL and reported vestibular hypofunction in 75%, with 47% demonstrating bilateral vestibular areflexia. [Ribari 1999]

Studies in children with hearing loss have found that the incidence of vestibular hypofunction ranges from 49-95% of those tested. Horak and colleagues compared 30 hearing impaired children and 15 learning-disabled children to a group of 54 normal controls using both vestibular and motor testing. Two-thirds of hearing impaired children had abnormal vestibulo-ocular reflexes compared to one-fifth of learning disabled children and seven percent of normal controls. Normal controls scored in the 84th percentile on motor testing compared to 29th percentile for hearing impaired children with vestibular loss and 44th percentile for hearing impaired children without vestibular loss. Of note, the difference in motor scores between hearing impaired children and normal controls was entirely attributable to the balance subset of motor testing scores, all other areas tested, such as running speed and strength, fell within the normal range for all children tested. [Horak 1988] In another study examining the role of vestibular dysfunction in learning disability, children with hearing loss and vestibular hypofunction were found to have poorer reading acuity scores than peers with normal vestibular function (regardless of hearing status). An especially large difference was noted in dynamic visual acuity, during which the subjects head is passively moved side-to side during testing. These findings suggest that a component of learning disabilities in the context of hearing loss may be due to deficiencies in reading acuity associated with vestibular dysfunction. [Braswell 2006]

Kaga used a series of interesting cases to describe the motor development of children with congenital and acquired bilateral vestibular losses. In general, patients with congenital bilateral vestibular loss showed good compensation for the loss, and though developmental milestones were somewhat delayed compared to age-matched controls, acquisition of demanding motor skills was eventually achieved. In one case of labyrinthine agenesis, running, hopping on one foot with eyes closed and gymnastics were possible at age 6; in another jumping rope, ice skating, and bicycling were possible at age 12. Outcomes were markedly worse in patients with concomitant mental retardation. Developmental delays were worse in patients with acquired bilateral vestibular loss; however, adequate function was generally reacquired if the insult occurred prior to 18 months of age. In a case of acquired vestibular loss due to meningitis at age 11 months, the patient had previously developed head control, crawling, sitting, standing, and walking. All gross-motor skills except crawling were lost, and subsequently reacquired by age 26 months. Acquired vestibular losses at an older age were associated with failure to develop more demanding gross-motor skills such as standing on one foot, bicycle riding, and swimming. [Kaga 1999]

2. Cochlear Implantation and Vestibular Function

Much study has focused recently on vestibular function in children receiving cochlear implants (CI). Of particular concern is the risk of bilateral vestibular loss resulting from bilateral cochlear implantation. As evidence of improved sound localization and hearing-in-noise with bilateral CI increases [Das 2005], more children are receiving bilateral CI, with many centers recommending this as standard-of-care in appropriate cases. Numerous studies in adults have demonstrated a quantitative decrease in vestibular function following unilateral CI. Buchman summarized fourteen studies describing the effect of unilateral CI on the caloric response. When combined, 71 of 186 patients (38%) had a reduced caloric response. However, conflicting conclusions have been reached with improved, worsened, or unchanged patient perception of balance function and dizziness on qualitative or quality of life measures. [Bonnucci 2008, Buchman 2004, Filipo 2006, Vibert 2001] Buchman's own data show 29% of patients experiencing an ipsilateral reduction in total caloric response of 21 degrees per second or greater after unilateral CI. These patients also had measureable worsening of vestibular function demonstrated on rotational chair testing and computerized dynamic posturography. Nonetheless, scores on the *Dizziness Handicap Inventory*, a validated quality of life questionnaire, were significantly improved one year postoperatively. Furthermore, there was a significant improvement in objective measures of postural stability. Device activation in music also appeared to have a positive effect on postural stability. [Buchman 2004]

Fewer studies have examined the impact of unilateral CI on vestibular function in children. Jacot and colleagues examined 224 children with profound SNHL prior to unilateral CI and found 50% to have abnormal bilateral vestibular function. Of the patients with existing vestibular function prior to CI, 70% experienced a post-CI worsening of vestibular function; 10% of patients developed complete ipsilateral vestibular areflexia as evaluated by clinical exam, ENG with rotational testing, bithermal caloric testing, and VEMP. [Jacot 2009] Licameli and colleagues investigated the prevalence and severity of vestibular impairment in two groups of children with CI. The first group consisted of 42 patients who had previously undergone CI and were being evaluated for a contralateral implant. These patients underwent testing of the vestibulo-ocular reflex (VOR), computerized dynamic posturography (CDP), and VEMP testing. 52% had abnormal VOR, 39% had abnormal CDP, and 80% had reduced or absent VEMP in the ipsilateral ear. The second group included 19 CI candidates (unilateral) who were prospectively evaluated for the outcome of VEMP testing pre- and post-implantation. 17 patients (89%) had VEMP responses preoperatively. After implantation, 14 of these patients experienced disappearance of VEMP or reduction of VEMP (measured by increased threshold or decreased amplitude) compared with their preoperative VEMP. [Licameli 2009] Cushing and colleagues performed caloric, rotational, and VEMP testing in addition to motor proficiency testing in a group of 40 children with unilateral CI. Abnormal horizontal semicircular canal function in response to caloric testing was found in 50% of patients, and in 38% of patients in response to rotation. Absent saccular function was demonstrated in 38% of patients, half of whom had bilaterally absent VEMP. Age standardized balance abilities were significantly diminished in the study population compared to normal hearing controls, and correlated best with rotational testing. [Cushing 2008]

Based on these findings, all of the above investigators advocate for vestibular testing, when feasible, in any pediatric CI candidate prior to surgery. While no consensus has been reached on the ideal timing and extent of such testing, Jacot and colleagues suggest a clinical vestibular examination including the head thrust test, bithermal caloric testing, and VEMP. They further recommend that in the case of unilateral CI, the ear with poorer vestibular function should be chosen for implantation to minimize the potential impact of further vestibular loss. When bilateral CI is planned, it is recommended that simultaneous bilateral CI be avoided except in cases of hearing loss due to bacterial meningitis (which is typically followed by a rapid cochlear ossification, making the procedure technically challenging); instead the surgeries should be separated by a period of three months to allow compensation for any vestibular loss incurred. [Jacot 2009] To date, no studies have been published which compare balance and vestibular function before and after bilateral cochlear implantation or assess the long-term developmental consequences of bilateral cochlear implantation.

Conductive Hearing Loss

Otitis media is one of the most common diseases in infants and children. [Bluestone 2004] Acute otitis media (AOM) occurs at least once in up to 71% of children under 3 years of age and an episode of AOM is followed by persistent middle ear fluid (otitis media with effusion, OME) for at least four weeks in 60% of cases. [Teele 1980] While OME frequently follows an acute upper respiratory infection or an episode of AOM, its proximate cause is typically Eustachian tube dysfunction. In one study, children aged 2-6 examined monthly over a 2-year period were found to have a cumulative incidence of OME of up to 61%. [Casselbrant 1985] Treatment of OME includes medical or surgical interventions. Because the recurrence and persistence rates of middle ear effusion are high after medical therapy, insertion of tympanostomy tubes is the preferred treatment for recurrent or persistent middle ear effusion.

The principal effect of OME on hearing consists of a mild-to-moderate conductive hearing loss with an average threshold of 27dB. [Fria 1984] This degree of hearing loss may delay speech development and be associated with learning disabilities. In addition, Eustachian tube dysfunction with and without middle ear effusion is considered one of the most common cause of vestibular disturbances in children. [Balkany 1986, Busis 1976] Anecdotal evidence from parents suggests that children with OME often exhibit a high degree of movement disorganization and propensity for falls especially compared to their peers without middle ear disease. Parents further report that their children often begin to walk or become less clumsy after tympanostomy tube insertion. More recently, studies in children have produced evidence supporting both the notion that vestibular, balance and motor function may deteriorate in the setting of middle-ear effusion and that this deterioration is reversed with resolution of OME.

Merica studied 135 patients with vertigo and Eustachian tube obstruction and found this association to be a distinct clinical entity from other causes of vertigo. [Merica 1942] Cohen and colleagues evaluated 25 subjects aged 13–57 months with OME using the Peabody Developmental Motor Scales (PDMS), a standardized test of motor development. Parents were also administered questionnaires about their children's balance skills. Subjects with bilateral OME were significantly impaired compared to age-matched controls on balance, locomotion and total score. Parental perceptions of their children's balance correlated poorly with the test results. [Cohen 1997]

Children with otitis media may be more visually dependent as a result of the deterioration of vestibular function causing excessive reliance on other non-vestibular sensory cues to maintain balance. Furthermore, placement of tympanostomy tubes in children with otitis media has been shown to improve balance. Casselbrant and colleagues tested 41 children with OME using moving platform posturography before and after insertion of tympanostomy tubes. Compared to children with no ear disease, speed of sway was found to be higher in children with OM than in normal children. For children tested less than 30 days after insertion of tympanostomy tubes, the velocity for condition VI of the sensory organization test (movements of both platform and visual field are synchronized with patient sway) was significantly lower than before. Children who had fallen on initial trials were able to stand on these trials after insertion of tympanostomy tubes. [Casselbrant 1995] Golz and colleagues tested 136 children, 4 to 9 years of age, using electronystagmography and the Bruininks-Oseretsky Test of Motor Proficiency (BOTMP) before and after tube ventilation of the middle ear. Pathologic findings on either study were found in 58% of the children with chronic middle ear effusion, as compared with only 4% of healthy controls. Balance disturbances resolved in 96% of subjects after tympanostomy tube insertion. [Golz 1998] Hart and colleagues compared 19 four- to six-year-old children with OME scheduled for tympanostomy tube insertion to 14 matched controls using the PDMS and the BOTMP. The OME group demonstrated significantly lower performance in the balance subscales prior to tube insertion. While both otitis and control groups improved on repeat testing, a trend toward greater improvement in the otitis group on the PDMS and BOTMP (P = .056 and .097, respectively) was seen. [Hart 1998] Jones and colleagues compared 34 children with OME with 34 age- and gender-matched control children between the ages of 3 and 5 years. Body sway was measured in both groups at four month intervals. Balance, as measured by sway velocity and several other factors, was found to be significantly worse in children with OME compared to controls. The increased rate of body sway of children with OME returned to the normal range following tympanostomy tube insertion. [Jones 1990] Casselbrant and colleagues found that children aged three to nine years with OME had increased postural sway in response to moving visual scenes, compared to age- and gender-matched controls, with statistically significant differences noted at both tested frequencies of surround movement. [Casselbrant 1998] The above studies indicate that balance-related symptoms in young children may result from OME and that these symptoms often resolve after middle ear aeration returns to normal. In addition to postural control abnormalities, some studies have indicated that children with otitis media can have spontaneous and positional nystagmus, which resolves after tympanostomy tube insertion. [Golz 1991]

The pathophysiologic basis for the balance disturbance seen in children with otitis media is still unknown and further studies are required to determine the cause. Suggested etiologies include derangement of endolymphatic ion concentrations by exchange via the semi-permeable round window membrane, serous or toxic labyrinthitis, and transmission of negative middle ear pressures to the vestibule via the labyrinthine windows. [Schachern 1987, Goycoolea 1988, Carlborg 1992]

Other sequelae of Eustachian tube dysfunction and otitis media which result in conductive hearing loss in children include negative middle ear pressure, cholesteatoma, and ossicular abnormalities. The effect of these entities on balance and vestibular function is unknown.

Rehabilitation of Balance and Motor Skills in the Hearing Impaired Child

The detection of vestibular, motor, and balance dysfunction in hearing impaired children is particularly relevant in the context of rehabilitation. As described above, children with peripheral vestibular hypofunction in the setting of a normal central nervous system are likely to compensate well in most environments. Nevertheless, early identification of specific functional deficits can guide rehabilitative efforts. Even when such children have excellent motor skills, strength, and speed, they may be labeled clumsy when they fall or lose balance in conditions with poor or unreliable visual and proprioceptive inputs. [Horak 88]

Rine and colleagues studied the effectiveness of exercise intervention on motor development in children with SNHL and vestibular loss. 21 children aged 3-8 years with bilateral vestibular impairment on rotary chair testing were divided into exercise and placebo groups. A statistically significant improvement in motor development was demonstrated in the intervention group, but not in the control group. Control patients were subsequently treated with exercise intervention, and demonstrated a comparable improvement. [Rine 2004] In a preliminary study involving two subjects with SNHL and bilateral vestibular hypofunction, an exercise program using head movements in the setting of complex backgrounds was employed. Both subjects showed improvement in critical print size nearing clinical significance. One subject had an improved dynamic visual acuity score. [Braswell 2006]

With the exception of the above studies, the literature is relatively deficient on the potential for various interventions to improve balance and motor development in SNHL patients with vestibular loss and impaired motor development. This remains a field with exciting potential for growth.

Conclusion

Numerous clinical studies have addressed the issue of balance and vestibular function in children with hearing loss. Balance is often impaired in children with otitis media, which is associated with a conductive hearing loss, and reversal of otitis media either spontaneously or by surgical intervention can improve this deficit. Significant evidence demonstrates the association of balance disturbances, vestibular dysfunction, and motor delay in children with sensorineural hearing loss. It is important to assess vestibular function in infants and young children with SNHL and delayed motor development, as abnormalities in the vestibular system may be the cause of developmental delay. In these cases, appropriate intervention and rehabilitation may lead to improvement in motor skills and development. Vestibular function testing can be beneficial in the cochlear implant candidate by increasing awareness of potential risks to normal motor development. Further research is needed to demonstrate the full potential of rehabilitation in this important group.

References

[1]   USPSTF. Universal screening for hearing loss in newborns: US Preventive Services Task Force recommendation statement. *Pediatrics* 2008;122(1):143-8.

[2]   Arnvig J. Vestibular function in deafness and severe hardness of hearing. *Acta Oto-Laryngologica* 1955;45(4):283-8.

[3]   Sandberg LE, Terkildsen K. CALORIC TESTS IN DEAF CHILDREN. *Archives of Otolaryngology* 1965;81:350-4.

[4]   Krause E, Louza JP, Hempel JM, Wechtenbruch J, Rader T, Gurkov R. Prevalence and characteristics of preoperative balance disorders in cochlear implant candidates. *Annals of Otology, Rhinology & Laryngology* 2008;117(10):764-8.

[5]   Krause E, Wechtenbruch J, Rader T, Gurkov R. Influence of cochlear implantation on sacculus function. *Otolaryngology - Head & Neck Surgery* 2009;140(1):108-113.

[6]   Ribari O, Kustel M, Szirmai A, Repassy G. Cochlear implantation influences contralateral hearing and vestibular responsiveness. *Acta Oto-Laryngologica* 1999;119(2):225-8.

[7]   Horak F, Shumway-Cook A, Black FO. Are vestibular deficits responsible for developmental disorders in children? *Insights in Otolaryngology* 1988;3(3).

[8]   Braswell J, Rine RM. Evidence that vestibular hypofunction affects reading acuity in children. *International Journal of Pediatric Otorhinolaryngology* 2006;70(11):1957-65.

[9]   Kaga K. Vestibular compensation in infants and children with congenital and acquired vestibular loss in both ears. *International Journal of Pediatric Otorhinolaryngology* 1999;49(3):215-24.

[10] Das S, Buchman CA. *Bilateral cochlear implantation: current concepts. Current Opinion in Otolaryngology & Head & Neck Surgery* 2005;13(5):290-3.

[11] Bonucci AS, Costa Filho OA, Mariotto LD, Amantini RC, Alvarenga Kde F. Vestibular function in cochlear implant users. *Revista Brasileira de Otorrinolaringologia* 2008;74(2):273-8.

[12] Buchman CA, Joy J, Hodges A, Telischi FF, Balkany TJ. Vestibular effects of cochlear implantation. *Laryngoscope* 2004;114(10 Pt 2 Suppl 103):1-22.

[13] Filipo R, Patrizi M, La Gamma R, D'Elia C, La Rosa G, Barbara M. Vestibular impairment and cochlear implantation. *Acta Oto-Laryngologica* 2006;126(12):1266-74.

[14] Vibert D, Hausler R, Kompis M, Vischer M. Vestibular function in patients with cochlear implantation. *Acta Oto-Laryngologica Supplement* 2001;545:29-34.

[15] Jacot E, Van Den Abbeele T, Debre HR, Wiener-Vacher SR. Vestibular impairments pre- and post-cochlear implant in children. *Int J Pediatr Otorhinolaryngol* 2009;73(2):209-17.

[16] Licameli G, Zhou G, Kenna MA. Disturbance of vestibular function attributable to cochlear implantation in children. *Laryngoscope* 2009;119(4):740-5.

[17] Cushing SL, Papsin BC, Rutka JA, James AL, Gordon KA. Evidence of vestibular and balance dysfunction in children with profound sensorineural hearing loss using cochlear implants. *Laryngoscope* 2008;118(10):1814-23.

[18] Bluestone CD. Studies in otitis media: Children's Hospital of Pittsburgh-University of Pittsburgh progress report--2004. *Laryngoscope* 2004;114(11 Pt 3 Suppl 105):1-26.

[19] Teele DW, Klein JO, Rosner BA. Epidemiology of otitis media in children. *Annals of Otology, Rhinology, & Laryngology - Supplement* 1980;89(3 Pt 2):5-6.

[20] Casselbrant ML, Brostoff LM, Cantekin EI, Flaherty MR, Doyle WJ, Bluestone CD, et al. Otitis media with effusion in preschool children. *Laryngoscope* 1985;95(4):428-36.

[21] Fria TJ, Cantekin EI, Eichler JA, et. al. The effect of otitis media with effusion ("secretory" otitis media) on hearing sensitivity in children. In: Lim D, Bluestone C, Klein J, et. al., editors. *Recent Advances in Otitis Media with Effusion.* Burlington, Ontario, Canada: BC Decker Inc; 1984. p. 320-324.

[22] Balkany TJ, Finkel RS. The dizzy child. Ear & Hearing 1986;7(3):138-42.

[23] Busis SN. Vertigo in children. *Pediatric Annals* 1976;5(8):478-81.

[24] Merica FW. Vertigo due to obstruction of the Eustachian tubes. *JAMA* 1942;118:1282-1284.

[25] Cohen H, Friedman EM, Lai D, Pellicer M, Duncan N, Sulek M. Balance in children with otitis media with effusion. *International Journal of Pediatric Otorhinolaryngology* 1997;42(2):107-15.

[26] Casselbrant ML, Furman JM, Rubenstein E, Mandel EM. Effect of otitis media on the vestibular system in children. *Annals of Otology, Rhinology & Laryngology* 1995;104(8):620-4.

[27] Golz A, Netzer A, Angel-Yeger B, Westerman ST, Gilbert LM, Joachims HZ. Effects of middle ear effusion on the vestibular system in children. *Otolaryngology - Head & Neck Surgery* 1998;119(6):695-9.

[28] Hart MC, Nichols DS, Butler EM, Barin K. Childhood imbalance and chronic otitis media with effusion: effect of tympanostomy tube insertion on standardized tests of balance and locomotion. *Laryngoscope* 1998;108(5):665-70.

[29] Jones NS, Radomskij P, Prichard AJ, Snashall SE. Imbalance and chronic secretory otitis media in children: effect of myringotomy and insertion of ventilation tubes on body sway. *Annals of Otology, Rhinology & Laryngology* 1990;99(6 Pt 1):477-81.

[30] Casselbrant ML, Redfern MS, Furman JM, Fall PA, Mandel EM. Visual-induced postural sway in children with and without otitis media. *Annals of Otology, Rhinology & Laryngology* 1998;107(5 Pt 1):401-5.

[31] Golz A, Westerman ST, Gilbert LM, Joachims HZ, Netzer A. Effect of middle ear effusion on the vestibular labyrinth. *Journal of Laryngology & Otology* 1991;105(12):987-9.

[32] Schachern PA, Paparella MM, Goycoolea MV, Duvall AJ, 3rd, Choo YB. The permeability of the round window membrane during otitis media. *Archives of Otolaryngology -- Head & Neck Surgery* 1987;113(6):625-9.

[33] Goycoolea MV, Muchow D, Schachern P. Experimental studies on round window structure: function and permeability. *Laryngoscope* 1988;98(6 Pt 2 Suppl 44):1-20.

[34] Carlborg BI, Konradsson KS, Carlborg AH, Farmer JC, Jr., Densert O. Pressure transfer between the perilymph and the cerebrospinal fluid compartments in cats. *American Journal of Otology* 1992;13(1):41-8.

[35] Horak FB, Shumway-Cook A, Crowe TK, Black FO. Vestibular function and motor proficiency of children with impaired hearing, or with learning disability and motor impairments. *Developmental Medicine & Child Neurology* 1988;30(1):64-79.

[36] Rine RM, Braswell J, Fisher D, Joyce K, Kalar K, Shaffer M. Improvement of motor development and postural control following intervention in children with sensorineural hearing loss and vestibular impairment. *International Journal of Pediatric Otorhinolaryngology* 2004;68(9):1141-8.

[37] Braswell J, Rine RM. Preliminary evidence of improved gaze stability following exercise in two children with vestibular hypofunction. *International Journal of Pediatric Otorhinolaryngology* 2006;70(11):1967-73.

In: Neuroplasticity in the Auditory Brainstem   ISBN 978-1-61761-949-6
Editor: Angelo Salami, pp. 75-94   © 2011 Nova Science Publishers, Inc.

Chapter VI

The Effect of Brain Plasticity on the Results of Cochlear Implantation

Seung-Ha Oh

Department of Otorhinolaryngology, Seoul National University, Seoul South Korea

Abstract

Cochlear implantation is both highly effective and the only method available for the auditory rehabilitation of profoundly deaf patients. The implant transfers the extracted characteristics of speech sounds to each electrode and then stimulates the spiral ganglion. Despite this technical achievement, currently such devices cannot fully replicate the function of the human ear. Furthermore, outcomes are highly diverse among implantees and the factors that determine outcome have yet to be fully elucidated.

The results of cochlear implantation are determined by three factors: *Device, Environments,* and *Patient-associated factors.* Device-associated factors depend on the hardware and software used, such as the number of electrodes and the sound processing strategy. Device improvements continually enhance speech rehabilitation results, but technological progress usually takes decade. Environmental factors largely affect accessibility to post-surgical rehabilitation. Socioeconomic status, family cooperation, and educational setting are all environmental factors. Patient factors are associated with the anatomical and neurophysiological status of the auditory system of the implantee and have intrinsic effects on outcome. Such factors include 'age at deafness', 'age at operation', 'cause of deafness', and 'mode of communication prior to surgery'. The contributions made by device and environmental factors cannot be over emphasized, but even a thorough understanding of the effects of these factors would not allow precise prediction of CI outcome without considering patient-associated factors. Furthermore, the orchestration of the combined effects of these three factors is not fully understood.

Sensory maps within somatosensory, visual, and auditory systems in the brain are altered when associated peripheral sensory organs are damaged. For example, cortical structures deprived of their normal auditory sensory inputs can become responsive to the stimulation of other sensory modalities. This reorganization of cortical functions across different sensory systems, which is called cross-modal plasticity[1], has been demonstrated for activation of the auditory cortex via visual stimulation, such as lip reading [2] and sign language[3]. Since, it has not been determined how cross-modal plasticity in deaf patients influences the results of cochlear implantation,. analyses of brain cortical function in the pre-implantation deaf and of functional changes following cochlear implantation are required in order to understand outcome variability. A better understanding of relationship of brain function with later outcome may enable the development of customized rehabilitation strategies that maximize implant benefit on an individual basis. In this chapter, we discuss the implications of a series of human brain imaging studies, relying mainly on Positron Emission Tomography (PET), as well as supporting animal studies that employed a variety of approaches

1. The Importance of Brain Research in Deaf Patients

A patient is considered deaf when he or she becomes incapable of perceiving common speech sound despite the use of hearing aids, which is synonymous with a complete loss of hearing capacity. Deaf patients can be classified according to the onset of deafness in relation to language acquisition, that is, as either prelingually or postlingually deaf. In postlingually deaf patients who were previously capable of comprehending normal speech, the cortical resource for auditory language processing must have been fully developed. Therefore, their neural resources can presumably facilitate reconstitution of hearing capacity following cochlear implantation, resulting in relatively intact speech perception ability. In contrast, prelingually deaf patients face difficulties in learning language through cochlear implants and their outcomes can be diverse.

As has been shown by many studies, the outcome of cochlear implantation is difficult to foresee. In particular, evaluations of hearing capacity, cognitive function, and language capability are challenging in young prelingually deaf patients, which makes it even more difficult to analyze the validity of outcome predicting factors.

Several studies have been devoted to identifying the factors that affect outcome by analyzing speech perception results after surgery. Researchers have attempted to identify prognostic factors in the prelingually deaf by reviewing biographic data, such as age, duration of deafness, and numbers of electrodes. Currently, 'age at implantation' is considered to be the most influential factor. It has been reported that better results are obtained when surgery is undertaken at a younger age [4, 5]. In another study that compared five possible outcome predictors in 40 prelingually deaf patients implanted under the age of seven with speech perception ability at 5 years post-surgery, 'age at surgery' and 'communication mode used prior to surgery' were found to be significantly correlated with outcome. However, these two factors were found to account for only 43 percent of the correlation, which suggests that other factors also determine the outcome of cochlea implantation [6].

Considering the mechanism of cochlear implants, it has been suggested that a significant association exists between the number of spiral ganglion cells directly stimulated by electrodes and speech perception ability. Although animal experiments supported this theory [7], the results obtained are probably inapplicable in humans. In 2001, an autopsy study was undertaken to determine spiral ganglion cell numbers in eight cochlear implant users by performing histopathologic analyses of the temporal bone. Contrary to the expectation, the study failed to provesignificant correlation between spiral ganglion cell number and speech perception performance. Therefore, although once regarded as being less significant, it is now believed that the central auditory system, including the cerebral cortex, plays a more important role in governing outcome than the peripheral auditory system [8].

Research on the cerebral cortex in deaf patients is crucial to enable us to understand primary and secondary changes in central auditory function It is also likely that an improved understanding of this issue would facilitate the customized rehabilitation of patients following cochlear implantation.

2. Cross-Modal Plasticity

The sensory cortices of the brain are subdivided by sensory modality into regions that process visual, auditory, gustatory, olfactory, and somatosensory signals. When one peripheral sensory organ is compromised, the cortex that serves the lost organ becomes responsive to stimuli from other sensory organs. This recommitment of sensory cortices constitutes the definition of the phenomena known as Cross-Modal Plasticity [1].

A prime example is provided by a blind subject reading Braille, in which case the brain receives tactile stimuli, but the visual cortex responds to this somatosensory input and comprehends its meaning [9]. Such plasticity also occurs in the auditory cortex, which is used to process visual information during lip-reading [2] or sign-language [3].

However, little is known about the implications of cross-modal plasticity on cochlear implant outcome. Brain plasticity observed in a prelingually deaf patient who has received cochlear implant surgery can be attributed to several mechanisms such as developmental plasticity, deaf-induced plasticity, and plasticity subsequent to cochlear implantation. In particular, the plasticity that occurs as a consequence of surgery has two aspects, namely, the plasticity resulting from the introduction of auditory stimuli and that resulting from the acquisition of language [10].

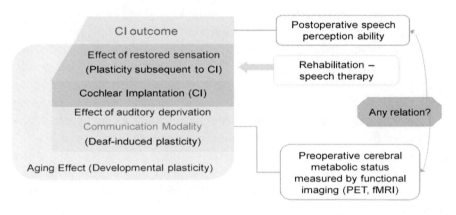

Figure 1. Potential influences of brain plasticity on the outcome of cochlear implantation (CI) in deaf children.

The results of cochlear implant surgery are presumably due to a conglomeration of such plasticities, with variations due to different contributions of each component of plasticity. If a congenitally deaf patient is implanted at age two, both developmental changes and deaf-induced plasticity that have been induced during these first two years of life would coexist with subsequent changes induced by rehabilitation. On the other hand, if a congenitally deaf subject received surgery at age seven, developmental and concomitant plasticity would be more seriously affected by central nervous system status prior to implant placement. Hence, it could be surmised that the effectiveness of surgery is likely to differ markedly in these two types of patients. Therefore, research on the correlation between cerebral plasticity before surgery and the ability to improve speech perception subsequently is crucial to our understanding of individual performance. (Figure 1)

3. Method Used to Evaluate Human Brain Function

Brain function can be investigated by numerous methods such as neuropsychologic analysis, electrophysiologic tests, and neuroimaging techniques. To understand auditory-linguistic function, various neuropsychologic tests probe speech and language function. Electrophysiologic testing includes the measurements of potentials evoked by various auditory stimuli. Functional imaging techniques, such as fMRI (functional MRI), diffusion tensor imaging, positron emission tomography, and magnetoencephalography have been used frequently in the field of brain science.

fMRI measures functional characteristics of the brain by detecting changes in blood oxygenation in specific areas. When a subject is given a task during scanning, blood flow to the targeted cortical area can be estimated by detecting alterations in image intensity, known as the BOLD (blood oxygenation level dependent) signal.

fMRI provides both anatomical and functional views of the brain with excellent spatial resolution and allows activities to be measured over seconds. Furthermore, because of its noninvasive and radiation-free nature, multiple scans can be performed, which allows changes reflecting learning to be examined over time. However, fMRI does not image neural activity, but rather vascular response to oxygen demand, which can both lag functional activation and extend beyond the activation period.

Diffusion tensor imaging (DTI) provides a means of evaluating anatomical connectivity and the strength of this connectivity *in vivo*. Diffusion tensor tractography provides anatomical evidence of connectivity between brain regions, and fractional anisotropy (FA) provides important parametric DTI images of the strengths of connections. In one DTI study, sensorineural hearing impaired patients demonstrated the abnormality in the central auditory pathway.   [11]. However, fMIR and DTI can only be applied to deaf patients prior to implant surgery; because the potential risk to the patient and damage to the device caused by the magnetic fields inherent to these methods make it impossible to analyze brain function after implantation.

Positron Emission Tomography (PET) can be performed to detect how much of the brain's fuels (oxygen and glucose) are being consumed in different regions. The radioactive entities $H_2^{15}O$ (water) and ^{18}F-FDG (fluorodeoxyglucose) both emit a positron, which collides with an electron to emit two gamma ray photons in opposite directions. These photons are detected and reconstructed to yield a brain image after performing a normalization procedure. $H_2^{15}O$ has a short half life and represents the blood distribution during image acquisition, as does fMRI. However, ^{18}F-FDG-PET provides information on metabolic rates, and image intensities are directly related to metabolic activities and synaptic densities in regions of interest (ROIs). Unlike fMRI, PET studies are possible even after implantation. However, the spatial and temporal resolutions of PET are markedly poorer than those of fMRI. Furthermore, PET introduces radiation hazards, and thus, studies on young children must be carefully monitored.

Magnetoencephalography (MEG) provides accurate measures of neuronal activity on a millisecond basis. The dendrites of neurons during synaptic transmission generate magnetic signals as well as electrical currents, and MEG measures the magnetic fields produced by electrical activity in the brain, by using an extremely sensitive device called a SQUID (superconducting quantum interference device). Unlike electroencephalography, MEG can be used to localize sources of activity, though its ability to do so is limited because MEG can only detect the magnetic fields generated by a large number of neurons. The technique is non-invasive, but it is expensive and requires a magnetically shielded room to cover the equipment from external magnetic signals, including the Earth's magnetic field.

The above-mentioned neuroimaging methods enable us to probe functional structures in the human brain and enable brain mapping. Probabilistic templates of the human brain will undoubtedly be useful clinically as well as for basic brain science research [12].

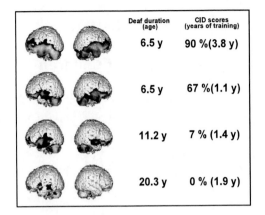

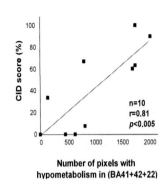

Figure 2. Correlation between auditory performance after cochlear implantation and pre-operative hypometabolism of the auditory cortex in prelingually deaf patients (Lee DS, Lee JS, Oh SH et al., Nature 2001).

Brain research in deaf subjects would help provide a better understanding of the changes of brain function consequent to auditory deprivation. Cochlear implantation affords a unique opportunity to restore sensory input in the profoundly deaf. Furthermore, research on brain functions associated with hearing deprivation and restoration can provide valuable information on cross-modal plasticity. Of the various functional neuroimaging techniques mentioned above, PET is a method of importance in patients using cochlear implants, and is the focus of the human research in this chapter.

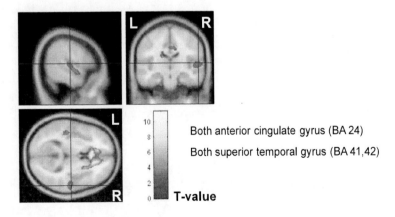

Figure 3. Brain areas showing a positive correlation between duration of deafness and glucose metabolism in postlingual deaf ($P<0.01$, uncorrected) (Lee JS, Lee DS, Oh SH, et al., J Nucl Med. 2003).

4. PET Studies in Deaf Patients

4.1. Cortical Metabolism in Prelingually Deaf Children

The term 'basal metabolism in the auditory cortex' refers to ambient activity in the region of interest. It might be presumed that metabolic activity in the regions related to auditory function is likely to be reduced in the deaf. In one of the early studies of auditory cortical metabolism, Ito et al. reported that in the deaf, cortical metabolism is reduced and this reduction increases with duration of hearing loss [13]. On the other hand, Catalan-Ahumada et al. reported that cortical metabolism is elevated in deaf subjects[14]Although the same FDG-PET method was used in these two studies, the patient populations and statistical methods were different Accordingly, further study was required to determine the nature of auditory cortical metabolic activity in the deaf. Thus we performed resting FDG-PET in 15 prelingually deaf patients and 17 normal hearing adults, and by using SPM (statistical parametric mapping; http://www.fil.ion.ucl.ac.uk/spm/), we compared cortical metabolism in Brodmann areas (BA) 41, 42, and 22) between these groups. We found that basal metabolism in the auditory related cortices of deaf subjects was lower than in normal subjects, but metabolic activity in the deaf increased up to the levels of normal controls when the duration of deafness was prolonged [15]. This recovery of auditory cortical metabolism in the absence of auditory stimulation is of considerable interest. Furthermore, the duration of deafness is inversely associated with open set speech perception ability (K-CID) following cochlear implantation. In this study, we proposed that this recovery is the result of cross-modal plasticity between the auditory and other sensory cortices, and that degree of cross-modal plasticity probably affects the postoperative development of auditory language. Consequently, this study suggests the prognostic importance of cross-modal plasticity in cochlear implant recipients (Figure 2). However, we were unable to recruit age-matched controls for ethical reasons, and thus, the possibility remains that the observed differences were caused by age differences.

4.2. Cortical Metabolism in Postlingually Deaf Adults

The issue as to whether cerebral plasticity exists in the adult brain is controversial. In one adult animal study, unilateral deafness was found to induce a reorganization of frequency rearrangements in the auditory cortex [16]. In the mature occipital cortex of blind individuals, a cross modal neural reorganization was also proposed to be exist [17, 18]. Furthermore, adult tinnitus patients were found to show a marked shift in the cortical representation of tinnitus frequency into an area adjacent to the expected tonotopic location, which suggests that plastic alterations occur in the auditory cortex [19]. In general, longer periods of deafness have been associated with poorer speech performance in postlingually deaf implantees. These findings support the possibility of auditory plasticity in the deaf adult brain [20, 21].

To investigate whether neuroplasticity exists in adults with postlingual deafness, we compared cerebral glucose metabolism measured by ^{18}F-FDG brain PET in 9 postlingually deaf patients with those of 9 age- and sex-matched healthy controls. The deaf group showed decreased metabolism in the anterior cingulate gyrus (BA24) and superior temporal gyri (BA41, BA42), and metabolic recovery in both areas was found to be significantly ($P = 0.005$) and positively correlated with deafness duration. However, we failed to demonstrate that metabolism in the adult auditory cortex is related to functional recovery (Figure 3) [22]. Further studies are required to ascertain whether metabolic recovery is associated with a rearrangement of cerebral function and whether this plasticity directly affects spoken word recognition following CI.

4.3. The Association between Cortical Metabolism and Post-implant Speech Perception in the Prelingually Deaf

Because the results of cochlear implantation in the prelingually deaf are variable, it is important to better understand the reasons for and patterns of cortical changes in the deaf. As individual variation of CI outcome was shown to be very widely among 5 to 7 year olds in our previous study [23], we tried to identify cortical areas related to postoperative speech perception in this age group. Patients who underwent cochlear implantation between 5 and 7 1/2 years of age and who were followed for more than 2 years were divided into 'good' and 'poor' groups based on results of speech perception test at 2 years post-CI. Pre-operative FDG-PET images of these two groups were then compared. It was found that the good group showed greater metabolism in the left posterior dorsolateral prefrontal gyrus (BA9) and right frontal pole (BA10), whereas the poor group showed greater metabolism in bilateral fusiform regions and in the right inferior occipital region. In view of the fact that BA9 and BA10 are involved in working memory function and/or judgment/decision making [24, 25], these results suggest that metabolism related to higher cognitive function and working memory must be secure as a functional prerequisite of a good speech perception result. On the other hand, increased metabolism in the fusiform area is associated with the ventral visual pathway ("what" pathway)[26, 27]. Accordingly, these findings indicate that if a prelingually deaf child relies more on the ventral visual pathway during spontaneous behavior, he or she will show less improvement in language acquisition even after successful implantation and concentrated rehabilitation (Figure 4) [28].

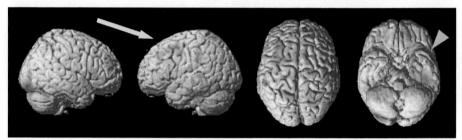

Figure 4. Brain areas with significant group differences in deaf children 5 to 7 years old. Higher metabolic activity (yellow arrow) and lower activity (arrow head) in the GOOD group relative to the POOR group. (Lee HJ, Kang E, Oh SH, et al., Hea Res. 2005).

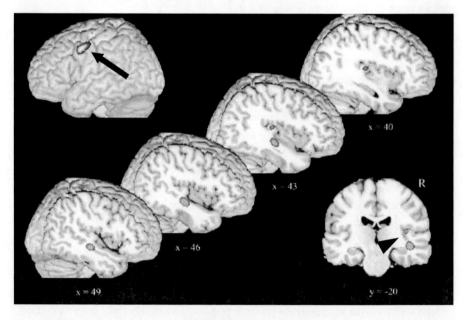

Figure 5. Brain regions showing correlations between brain metabolism and speech perception score. Areas of positive correlation are marked in hot color (long arrow) and those of negative correlation are marked in cold color (arrowhead). (Lee HJ, Giraud AL, Kang E et al., Cerebral Cortex 2007).

In our follow-up studies, we investigated whether the above phenomenon is present in deaf children of all age ranges. Accordingly, we correlated preoperative glucose metabolism measured by F-18-FDG-PET with individual speech perception performance assessed 3 years after implantation in 22 prelingually deaf children aged between 1 and 11 years. Analysis revealed that age at implantation was positively correlated with increased activity in the right superior temporal gyrus. When we adjusted for the comfounding effect of age at implantation, speech scores were found to be associated with decreased metabolic activity in the right Heschl's gyrus and posterior superior temporal sulcus. As in the former study on 5-7 year old children, metabolism in the left prefrontal area was found to be significantly associated with better speech perception ability, which again implies the importance of higher cognitive function for better outcomes, regardless of age at implantation. Conversely, metabolism in ventral areas of the brain was found to be negatively correlated with speech perception results, which suggests that greater dependency on visual function subserved by the occipito-temporal region due to auditory deprivation may interfere with the acquisition of auditory language after surgery (Figure 5) [29].

These results suggest that measures of cortical metabolism can be related to postoperative speech perception ability, and support the interesting notion that the use of certain cerebral regions as a compensatory modality can affect postoperative rehabilitation. However, this study could show only metabolic changes in the cerebral cortex , and thus further studies on the other functional changes are required.

4.4. Changes in Cortical Metabolism after Cochlear Implantation

In one study of 8 CI patients, we compared F-18-FDG-PET results before and after cochlear implant surgery. An increase of glucose metabolism was identified in the bilateral ventral posteromedial thalamus and the posterior cingulate gyrus. However, it should be determined whether these changes in metabolism might have been caused by a developmental effect. The middle occipito-temporal junction (hMT/V5) and the posterior inferior temporal region (BA 21/37) in the left hemisphere showed increases of glucose metabolism and these changes were found to be significantly associated with better speech perception ability. Therefore, the occipito-temporal junctional area in the left hemisphere appears to be important for speech development after implant surgery. These results mean that brain plasticity after surgery likely plays a role in learning language, allowing the use of new incoming auditory sensations in synchrony with visual cues (e.g., lip reading) (Figure 6) [30].

Another study also produced direct evidence of functional changes after cochlear implant surgery. Giraud et al. reported that the activities of the auditory and early visual cortices (V1/V2) increase in concert with rehabilitation duration in postlingually deaf adult patients. Thus, there appears to be a type of auditory-visual coordination that enables visual cues to compensate for incomplete auditory information from a cochlear implant, which in turn suggests a functional association between auditory and visual systems [31].

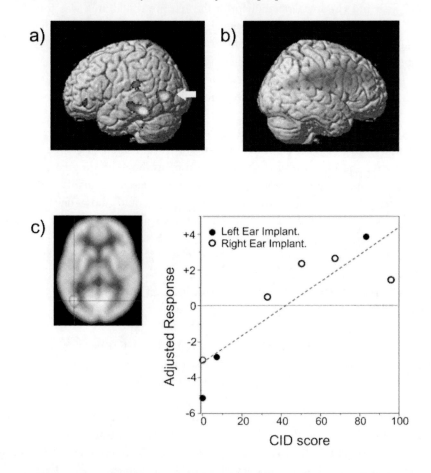

Figure 6. Brain regions with a positive (a) and negative (b) correlation between the FDG-uptake changes and the CID scores c) Greater increase of glucose metabolism in the left middle occipito-temporal junction (V5, MT) following CI was found to be correlated with greater improvement of auditory performance. (Kang E et al., Neuroimage 2004).

5. Changes in Cognitive Function in Deaf Patients

It has been reported that cortical metabolism related to cognitive function and working memory is a significant predictor of implantation language development [28, 29]. Although some studies have already reported that working memory and cognitive function in postoperative implant patients are positively correlated with speech perception ability [32, 33], it seemed worth investigating whether cochlear implantation facilitates cognitive development. Consequently we administered a neuropsychological test battery to 17 deaf children (mean age, 7 yr 2 mo) before receiving cochlear implants, and reassessed the same children 6 months postoperatively. Children showed marked improvements in motor coordination and visual organization abilities, and nonverbal cognitive functions and working memory were markedly improved despite the lack of language ability improvement [34]. The relatively small sample size and the absence of a control group precluded firm conclusions, but this study did provide preliminary data regarding the prediction of outcome based on systematic assessments of cognitive functions. Nevertheless, more comprehensive, prospective, and long-term comparative research is required on the relations between auditory verbal ability and cognitive function and working memory with a view toward providing evidence regarding clinically relevant indicators.

6. Studies Using Deaf Animal Models

6.1. Changes in Auditory Cortex Metabolism in the White Rat Model

A previous study discovered that metabolism in the auditory cortex is lower in prelingually deaf patients than in normal controls[15]. However, the effect of maturation was not ruled out because ethical considerations prevented the recruitment of an age-matched control group. To compensate for this experimental shortcoming, an animal study was conducted using an age-matched control group. A deaf model was created by ablating the inner ears of white rats bilaterally within 2 weeks of birth, and cerebral cortical metabolism was gauged by measuring 2 DG (2-deoxyglucose) intensity. Auditory cortical metabolism was found to diminish 2-4 weeks after ablation and then to recover gradually.

However, cortical metabolism failed to surpass that of the normal group at any age, which is wholly in-line with observations in the human (Figure 7) [35]. Because animals seem to lack a capacity for language development, this observed reduction and recovery of auditory cortex metabolism suggests that the plasticity observed in deaf models is not confined to language acquisition. This was verified by PET in prelingually deaf children, for whom within the auditory cortex region, the area associated with duration of deafness is separated from the area correlated with speech perception. [29]. Furthermore, the notion that deafness *per se* can cause cross-plasticity in the lower-level auditory cortex has been demonstrated by observing auditory cortex activation after stimulating visual movement in congenitally deaf patients [36].

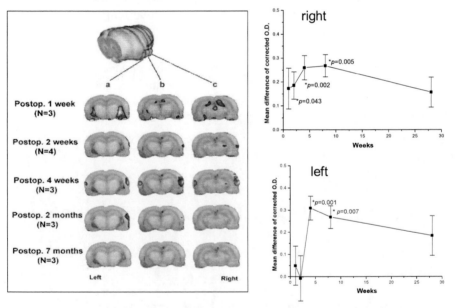

Figure 7. 3-D voxel-wise statistical analysis. The changes in the mean difference of the corrected optical density (OD) of right and left auditory cortex. (Ahn SH et al., Hear Res 2004).

6.2. Molecular Changes in the Auditory Cortex of a Deaf White Rat Model

Relatively little is known about biologic changes at the molecular level in the auditory cortex triggered by deafness. It is crucial to identify molecular changes related to brain plasticity, because this would contribute to an understanding of the mechanisms that underlie plastic change in the auditory cortex following hearing loss. Using the deaf rat model mentioned above, we used DNA microarrays to analyze differential gene expressions in the primary auditory cortex. We observed expressional changes in immediate early genes *(Egr1 , 2, 3, 4, c-fos , etc.)*, neural plasticity related genes *(Arc, Syngr1 , Bdnf , etc.)*, and neurotransmission related genes *(Gabra5, Chrnb3, Chrne, etc.)*. Further studies are warranted to elucidate the roles of these genes in the context of cortical development and plasticity[37]. In addition, in an attempt to identify the genes responsible for postlingual deafness, we performed a similar study using adult rats and Affymetrix GeneChips. It was found that the gene groups related to neural damage, apoptosis, tissue remodeling, and neural activity were modulated. (Data not shown, paper in preparation)

(a) (b)

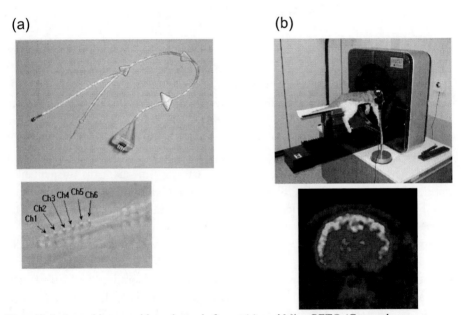

Figure 8. 6-channel intra-cochlear electrode for cat (a), and MicroPET® (Concord Microsystems Inc., Tenn. USA) for cat brain study (b).

6.3. Electrophysiologic and Metabolic Changes in the Auditory Cortex in a Deaf Cat Model

Cats have been extensively used in electrophysiological research of the cerebral cortex. Electrophysiologic studies in a deaf cat model using cochlear implantation should enable us to investigate the functional change of brain with respect to duration of deafness [38]. Recently, we developed a 3D voxel-based procedure for analyzing 2-deoxy-2-[18F]fluro-D-glucose-positron emission tomographic images of the cat brain, which showed high localization accuracy and specificity[39]. A longitudinal assessment of bilateral deafened cats showed a decrease and a recovery of metabolism in the auditory cortex which is similar to the human [40]. In the future, multi-channel cochlear implants and serial PET scan in the cat will enable more precise comparisons of functional imaging and electrophysiological findings. (Figure 8)

7. Summary and Future Research Directions

The aforementioned studies demonstrate that cross-plasticity in the auditory cortices of deaf patients plays an important role in the recovery of auditory language after cochlear implantation. Using FDG-PET, poor postoperative auditory language performance has been found to be associated with high levels of preoperative glucose metabolism in the high-level visual information processing region of the ventral visual pathway, which suggests that auditory language development after cochlear implantation is likely to be impeded if dependence on certain types of visual compensatory mechanisms are enhanced during the deaf period. On the other hand, children with good postoperative auditory language performance showed high levels of glucose metabolism in the dorsal visual pathway, indicating a higher visual spatial function. An improvement in speech perception has been found to be significantly correlated with increase of glucose metabolism at the occipito-temporal junction, which emphasizes the significance of comprehensive collaboration and subsequent mutual plasticity between the visual and auditory cortices. However, the PET studies conducted to date only provide indirect evidence of plasticity based on measures of resting state glucose metabolism. Future studies should focus on the functional confirmation of audio-visual cross-modal plasticity, and anatomical and functional evidence of audio-visual collaboration should be provided by DTI and other functional brain imaging modalities ($H_2^{15}O$-PET, etc).

We will continue to analyze high-level cognitive functions managed by the prefrontal lobe in congenitally deaf children deprived of auditory stimulation during the developmental period of the brain in an effort to identify the factors affecting postoperative development of auditory language.

Conclusion

Cochlear implantation is the only effective surgical method of rehabilitation in deaf patients, but the great variation in postoperative results observed has suggests a critical involvement of brain function. Furthermore, cortical plasticity, especially that involving audio-visual collaboration, has been shown to influence improvement of speech recognition ability following CI. We believe that the available functional imaging methods are capable of allowing cross-plasticity in the cerebral cortex and its functional meaning to be comprehended.

If individual characteristics of auditory-visual integration function are elucidated and effective individual rehabilitation programs devised, the benefit of cochlear implantation could be maximized. Finally, we emphasize that the importance of high-level cognitive function should not be underestimated, because it is required to learn to understand CI-mediated speech during the rehabilitation period.

Acknowledgments

This work was supported by grants from the Ministry of Education, Science, and Technology (No. 2009-0093890). The author appreciates the collaboration of the Department of Otorhinolaryngology (CS Kim, HJ Lee, JJ Song, and MH Park), the Department of Nuclear Medicine (DS Lee, JS Lee, and HJ Kang), and the Department of Neuropsychiatry (MS Shin) at Seoul National University College of Medicine.

The author also thanks Charles Limb, E Kang and HJ Lee for their comments on the manuscript and Robert Oh for editorial assistance.

References

[1]   Rauschecker, J.P., *Compensatory plasticity and sensory substitution in the cerebral cortex.* Trends Neurosci, 1995. 18(1): p. 36-43.

[2]   Calvert, G.A., et al., *Activation of auditory cortex during silent lipreading.* Science, 1997. 276(5312): p. 593-6.

[3]   Nishimura, H., et al., *Sign language 'heard' in the auditory cortex.* Nature, 1999. 397(6715): p. 116.

[4]   Nikolopoulos, T.P., G.M. O'Donoghue, and S. Archbold, *Age at implantation: its importance in pediatric cochlear implantation.* Laryngoscope, 1999. 109(4): p. 595-9.

[5]   Hassanzadeh, M., et al., *Effect of intermittent lighting schedules during the natural scotoperiod on T(3)-induced ascites in broiler chickens.* Avian Pathol, 2000. 29(5): p. 433-9.

[6]   O'Donoghue, G.M., T.P. Nikolopoulos, and S.M. Archbold, *Determinants of speech perception in children after cochlear implantation.* Lancet, 2000. 356(9228): p. 466-8.

[7]   Miller, A.L., *Effects of chronic stimulation on auditory nerve survival in ototoxically deafened animals.* Hear Res, 2001. 151(1-2): p. 1-14.

[8]   Nadol, J.B., Jr., et al., *Histopathology of cochlear implants in humans.* Ann Otol Rhinol Laryngol, 2001. 110(9): p. 883-91.

[9]   Sadato, N., et al., *Activation of the primary visual cortex by Braille reading in blind subjects.* Nature, 1996. 380(6574): p. 526-8.

[10]   Giraud, A.L., E. Truy, and R. Frackowiak, *Imaging plasticity in cochlear implant patients.* Audiol Neurootol, 2001. 6(6): p. 381-93.

[11]   Chang, Y., et al., *Auditory neural pathway evaluation on sensorineural hearing loss using diffusion tensor imaging.* Neuroreport, 2004. 15(11): p. 1699-703.

[12]   Lee, J.S., et al., *Development of Korean standard brain templates.* J Korean Med Sci, 2005. 20(3): p. 483-8.

[13]   Ito, J., et al., *Positron emission tomography of auditory sensation in deaf patients and patients with cochlear implants.* Ann Otol Rhinol Laryngol, 1993. 102(10): p. 797-801.

[14]   Catalan-Ahumada, M., et al., *High metabolic activity demonstrated by positron emission tomography in human auditory cortex in case of deafness of early onset.* Brain Res, 1993. 623(2): p. 287-92.

[15]   Lee, D.S., et al., *Cross-modal plasticity and cochlear implants.* Nature, 2001. 409(6817): p. 149-50.

[16]   Irvine, D.R., R. Rajan, and M. Brown, *Injury- and use-related plasticity in adult auditory cortex.* Audiol Neurootol, 2001. 6(4): p. 192-5.

[17]   Kujala, T., et al., *Electrophysiological evidence for cross-modal plasticity in humans with early- and late-onset blindness.* Psychophysiology, 1997. 34(2): p. 213-6.

[18]   Kujala, T., K. Alho, and R. Naatanen, *Cross-modal reorganization of human cortical functions.* Trends Neurosci, 2000. 23(3): p. 115-20.

[19]   Muhlnickel, W., et al., *Reorganization of auditory cortex in tinnitus.* Proc Natl Acad Sci U S A, 1998. 95(17): p. 10340-3.

[20]   Blamey, P., et al., *Factors affecting auditory performance of postlinguistically deaf adults using cochlear implants.* Audiol Neurootol, 1996. 1(5): p. 293-306.

[21] Proops, D.W., et al., *Outcomes from adult implantation, the first 100 patients.* J Laryngol Otol Suppl, 1999. 24: p. 5-13.

[22] Lee, J.S., et al., *PET evidence of neuroplasticity in adult auditory cortex of postlingual deafness.* J Nucl Med, 2003. 44(9): p. 1435-9.

[23] Oh, S.H., et al., *Speech perception after cochlear implantation over a 4-year time period.* Acta Otolaryngol, 2003. 123(2): p. 148-53.

[24] Owen, A.M., et al., *Planning and spatial working memory: a positron emission tomography study in humans.* Eur J Neurosci, 1996. 8(2): p. 353-64.

[25] Kammer, T., et al., *Functional MR imaging of the prefrontal cortex: specific activation in a working memory task.* Magn Reson Imaging, 1997. 15(8): p. 879-89.

[26] Ungerleider, L.G. and J.V. Haxby, *'What' and 'where' in the human brain.* Curr Opin Neurobiol, 1994. 4(2): p. 157-65.

[27] Ishai, A., et al., *Distributed representation of objects in the human ventral visual pathway.* Proc Natl Acad Sci U S A, 1999. 96(16): p. 9379-84.

[28] Lee, H.J., et al., *Preoperative differences of cerebral metabolism relate to the outcome of cochlear implants in congenitally deaf children.* Hear Res, 2005. 203(1-2): p. 2-9.

[29] Lee, H.J., et al., *Cortical activity at rest predicts cochlear implantation outcome.* Cereb Cortex, 2007. 17(4): p. 909-17.

[30] Kang, E., et al., *Neural changes associated with speech learning in deaf children following cochlear implantation.* Neuroimage, 2004. 22(3): p. 1173-81.

[31] Giraud, A.L., et al., *Cross-modal plasticity underpins language recovery after cochlear implantation.* Neuron, 2001. 30(3): p. 657-63.

[32] Pisoni, D.B. and A.E. Geers, *Working memory in deaf children with cochlear implants: correlations between digit span and measures of spoken language processing.* Ann Otol Rhinol Laryngol Suppl, 2000. 185: p. 92-3.

[33] Pisoni, D.B. and M. Cleary, *Measures of working memory span and verbal rehearsal speed in deaf children after cochlear implantation.* Ear Hear, 2003. 24(1 Suppl): p. 106S-20S.

[34] Shin, M.S., et al., *Comparison of cognitive function in deaf children between before and after cochlear implant.* Ear Hear, 2007. 28(2 Suppl): p. 22S-28S.

[35] Ahn, S.H., et al., *Changes of 2-deoxyglucose uptake in the rat auditory pathway after bilateral ablation of the cochlea.* Hear Res, 2004. 196(1-2): p. 33-8.

[36] Fine, I., et al., *Comparing the effects of auditory deprivation and sign language within the auditory and visual cortex.* J Cogn Neurosci, 2005. 17(10): p. 1621-37.

[37] Oh, S.H., C.S. Kim, and J.J. Song, *Gene expression and plasticity in the rat auditory cortex after bilateral cochlear ablation.* Acta Otolaryngol, 2007. 127(4): p. 341-50.

[38] Kral, A., et al., *Spatiotemporal patterns of cortical activity with bilateral cochlear implants in congenital deafness.* J Neurosci, 2009. 29(3): p. 811-27.

[39] Kim, J.S., et al., *Assessment of cerebral glucose metabolism in cat deafness model: strategies for improving the voxel-based statistical analysis for animal PET studies.* Mol Imaging Biol, 2008. 10(3): p. 154-61.

[40] Park, M.H., et al., *Cross-modal and compensatory plasticity in adult deafened cats: A longitudinal PET study.* Brain Res, 2010. 1354: p. 85-90.

In: Neuroplasticity in the Auditory Brainstem   ISBN 978-1-61761-949-6
Editor: Angelo Salami, pp. 95-118   © 2011 Nova Science Publishers, Inc.

Chapter VII

Pharmacology of New Drugs Used to Improve the Neuroplasticity of the Central Auditory Pathway

Antonella Sblendido and Giorgio Manini
Medical Department, Scharper Therapeutics, Sesto S. Giovanni (MI), Italy

Abstract

Following a peripheral damage localized in the cochlea or in the spiral ganglion, plastic changes occurring in the central auditory pathway may be adaptative, restoring as much as possible the normal hearing function, or maladaptative, perhaps leading to an imbalance of excitatory and inhibitory inputs and to the onset of tinnitus.

In the last years, scientific research has focused on identification of active principles that may direct neural network changes in an adaptative way.

Citicoline and coenzyme Q10 are two non-xenobiotic substances with an excellent safety profile, that benefit from complementary activities within the cells, in terms of protection from apoptotic cell death and support of structural and neurochemical changes involving synapses.

These molecules have demonstrated neuroprotective and neurorepairing activities in several in vitro and in vivo models of neurodegeneration or acute neuronal damage.

Even if clinical data in the audiological field are limited, their proprieties lay the foundations for the rational use of these compounds in hearing loss and tinnitus prevention.

Introduction

The term "neuroplasticity" refers to the ability of the central nervous system to reorganize its neural networks on the basis of novel experience.

This reorganization begins with changes in gene expression producing neuronal, glial or vascular modifications at the molecular, cellular and tissue levels. Ultimately, generation or elimination of synapses leads to modification of specific information processing function.

Following a peripheral damage localized in the cochlea or in the spiral ganglion, the plastic changes occurring in the central auditory pathway may be positive and adaptive, restoring as much as possible the normal hearing function. Alternatively, neuroplastic changes may be maladaptive, perhaps leading to an imbalance of excitatory and inhibitory inputs, that can clinically manifest through the phenomenon of tinnitus.

In the last years, great efforts have been made to identify active principles that may to influence and direct neural networks changes in an adaptive way.

Among the substances with demonstrated neuroprotective and neurorepairing activities there are coenzyme Q10 and citicoline.

Coenzyme Q10

CoQ10 is a naturally occurring lipophilic compound belonging to a homologous series of compounds that share a common benzoquinone ring structure, but differ in the length of the isoprenoid side chain.

In humans and a few other mammalian species, the side chain is comprised of 10 isoprene units, hence it is called coenzyme Q10 (CoQ10) (Figure 1).

CoQ_{10} is similar to vitamin K in its chemical structure but it is not considered a vitamin because it is synthesized in the body. The chemical nomenclature of CoQ10 is 2,3-dimethoxy-5-methyl-6-decaprenyl-1,4-benzoquinone, that is in the trans configuration (natural).

CoQ10 is present in all tissues in varying amounts. The total body pool of CoQ10 is estimated to be approximately 0.5–1.5 g in a normal adult [1].

As a general rule, tissues with high-energy requirements or metabolic activity such as brain, heart, kidney, liver and muscle contain relatively high concentrations of CoQ10 [2]. Being a lipophilic molecule, the distribution of CoQ10 in tissues is related not only to its metabolic activity but also to its lipid content. Data on the subcellular distribution of CoQ10 show a large portion (40–50%) of CoQ10 localized in the mitochondrial inner membrane, with smaller amounts in the other organelles (endoplasmic reticulum, peroxisomes, lysosomes, and vesicles) and also in the cytosol [3].

CoQ10 has a fundamental role in cellular bioenergetics as a cofactor in the mitochondrial electron transport chain (respiratory chain) and is therefore essential for the production of ATP [4, 5].

It participates in the electron transport chain by carrying electrons from complex I (succinate–ubiquinone oxidoreductase) to complex III (ubiquinone–cytochrome c oxidoreductase).

Furthermore, CoQ10 in its reduced form as the hydroquinone (called ubiquinol) is a potent lipophilic antioxidant. It is well located in membranes in close proximity to the unsaturated lipid chains to act as a primary scavenger of free radicals [6].

In addition to direct antioxidant radical scavenging, the quinol can rescue tocopheryl radicals produced by reaction with lipid or oxygen radicals by direct reduction back to tocopherol [7].

The efficiency of absorption of orally administered CoQ10 is poor because of its insolubility in water, limited solubility in lipids, and relatively high molecular weight (863 g/mol).

In one study in rats it was reported that only about 2–3% of orally-administered CoQ10 was absorbed [8]. As a general rule, higher the ingested dose lower the percent dose absorbed.

In the case of supplemental CoQ10 in the form of finished dosage forms, the absorption is also dependent on factors such as the nature of the formulation; solubilized formulations of CoQ10 have been shown to have enhanced bioavailability [9-11].

Basic Pharmacology and Toxicity

Being a lipophilic substance, the absorption of CoQ10 follows the same process as that of lipids in the gastrointestinal tract. The uptake mechanism for CoQ10 appears to be similar to that of vitamin E, another lipid-soluble nutrient. In the small intestine, secretions from the pancreas and bile facilitate emulsification and micelles formation that is required for fat absorption. No specific site along the small intestine has been identified for the absorption of CoQ10.

Comparably to vitamin E and other lipophilic substances, CoQ10 is first incorporated into chylomicrons following absorption and transported via the lymphatics into the circulation [12].

Data from rat studies indicate that CoQ10 is reduced to ubiquinol either during or following absorption in the intestine. This has been confirmed in a recent cell culture study using human Caco-2 cells [13].

Following absorption, ubiquinol first appears as a part of mesenteric triacylglycerol-rich lipoproteins. These particles are converted to chylomicron remnants in the circulation by lipoprotein lipase and then rapidly up taken by the liver, where CoQ10 is repackaged mostly into VLDL/LDL particles and rereleased into the circulation, in a comparable way as the handling of alpha tocopherol [14, 15]. HDL also contains a small amount of CoQ10.

Plasma CoQ10 concentrations are highly dependent on plasma lipoproteins [16]. Circulating CoQ10 redistributes among lipoproteins possibly to protect them from oxidation. About 95% of CoQ10 in the circulation exists in the reduced form , namely ubiquinol, in human subjects.

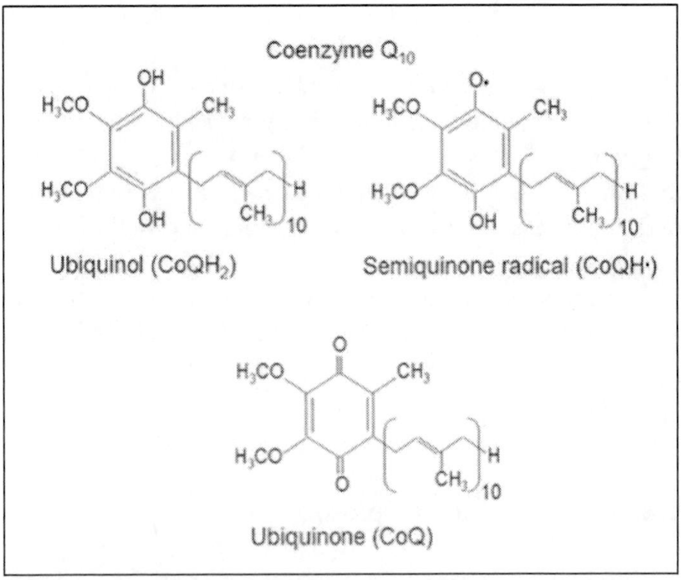

Figure 1. Chemical structure of CoQ10 as ubiquinone (oxidized form), ubiquinol (reduced form) and semiquinone radical.

A major portion of CoQ10 in tissues is in the reduced form, ubiquinol, with the exception of brain and lungs. This appears to be a reflection of increased oxidative stress in these two tissues.

In blood, about 95% of CoQ10 is in the reduced form [17, 18]. CoQ10 is also present in the cerebrospinal fluid mostly as ubiquinol at a very low concentration (about 9 pmol/l) as compared with plasma [19].

The efficiency of absorption of orally administered CoQ10 is poor because of its insolubility in water, limited solubility in lipids, and relatively large molecular weight. In one rat study, it was reported that only about 2–3% of orally-administered CoQ10 was absorbed [8]. As a general rule, higher the ingested dose lower the percent dose absorbed.

In the case of supplemental CoQ10 in the form of finished dosage forms, the absorption is also dependent on factors such as the nature of the formulation, whereas solubilized formulations of CoQ10 have been shown to have enhanced bioavailability [9, 10].

CoQ10 has an excellent safety record. The safety of high doses of orally-ingested CoQ10 over long periods is well documented in human subjects [20, 21] and also by chronic toxicity studies in animals [22]. The side effects reported in human studies are generally limited to mild gastrointestinal symptoms such as nausea and stomach upset seen in a small number of subjects. No adverse effects were observed with daily doses ranging from 600 to 1200 mg in two trials on Huntington's [23] and Parkinson's [24] diseases. More recent data document the safety and tolerability of CoQ10 at doses as high as 3000 mg a day in patients with Parkinson's disease [25] and amyotrophic lateral sclerosis [26].

Coenzyme Q10 and Neuroprotection

There is strong evidence showing involvement of reactive oxygen species (ROS) in the cascade of cochlear events that induces acoustic trauma [27].

The generation of ROS related to ischemia/reperfusion mechanism, glutamate excitotoxicity and endogenous antioxidant system reduction, leads to mitochondrial damage, membrane lipid peroxidation and eventually to apoptotic cell death [28].

In addition to being crucial for energy production and metabolic pathways, mitochondria also play a key role in integrating cell death stimuli and executing the apoptotic program.

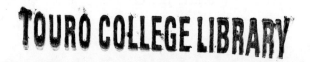

Apoptosis can be initiated through two major pathways: the extrinsic or membrane death receptor-dependent pathway and the intrinsic or mitochondrial pathway [29, 30].

The mitochondrial respiratory chain is a powerful source of reactive oxygen species (ROS), and oxidative stress triggers the opening of the mitochondrial permeability transition pores (PTP), causing the collapse of inner mitochondrial membrane potential and release of pro-apoptotic factors, as cytochrome c and/or apoptosis inducing factor (AIF) [31].

Given the major role of oxidative stress and mitochondrial dysfunction in the degenerative events following acoustic trauma or physiological aging, one would predict that agents that alleviate mitochondrial misfunction could be beneficial and exert neuroprotective effects.

Several bioenergetic agents that improve mitochondrial function, including coenzyme Q10, are being tested for their neuroprotective efficacy in neurodegenerative disorders.

Among them, CoQ10 is being tested in clinical trials for several neurodegenerative diseases characterized by oxidative stress and apoptosis (Parkinson, Huntington and amyotrophic lateral sclerosis) [32-38].

Coenzyme Q10 might exert positive effects in case of acoustic trauma through several mechanisms:

- *Free radical scavenging.* CoQ10 is a strong lipophilic antioxidant. It directly scavenges reactive oxygen species and can moreover regenerate other antioxidant molecules, as vitamin E [7].
- *Apoptosis inhibition.* CoQ10 also prevents apoptotic cell death by blocking Bax binding to mitochondria and by inhibiting activation of the mitochondrial permeability transition (MPT) [39-40]. CoQ10 is a cofactor of mitochondrial uncoupling proteins (UCP) and may also exert neuroprotective effects by activation of these proteins, leading to a reduction in mitochondrial-free radical generation [41, 42].
- *ATP production.* CoQ10 plays a key role in mitochondrial metabolism, leading to production of energy [4]. Neurosensorial cells, as inner and outer hair cells, and neurons composing central auditory pathway, exhibit a sustained oxidative metabolism and are therefore more vulnerable to oxidative stress.

The free radical scavenging and anti-apoptotic activity of CoQ10 might potentiate the bioprotective mechanism of inner or outer hair cells, resulting possibly in a minor mortality of these cells in response to oxidative stress, secondary to glutamate excitotossicity, ischemia/reperfusion events and cellular antioxidants decline due to aging.

The supporting action of oxidative metabolism performed by CoQ10 could supply inner and outer hair cells with the necessary amount of ATP to perform cell membrane and nucleic acids repair and to avoid apoptosis triggering.

Moreover plastic changes of neural networks composing central auditory pathways, which may follow a peripheral damage, require large amount of energy.

The outgrowth of axons and the active transport of various molecules from the cell body to the synapse and back requires energy. These processes include the polymerization of actin filaments and microtubules, interactions of actin and myosin, and the operation of "motor" proteins such as kinesin and dynein, which propel cargo along cytoskeletal tracks [43-46]. In a reciprocal manner, cytoskeletal proteins play a major role in controlling the location of mitochondria [47]. Mitochondria are actively transported in axons in both anterograde and retrograde directions. During development and regeneration, mitochondrial movements are associated with the outgrowth of axons [48].

As in other cells, neurons use adenosine triphosphate (ATP) as an energy source to drive biochemical processes involved in various cell functions, and produce reactive oxygen species (ROS) as "by products" of oxidative phosphorylation. However, the electrical excitability and structural and synaptic complexity of neurons present unusual demands upon cellular systems that produce ATP.

Mitochondria in axons and presynaptic terminals provide sources of ATP to drive the ion pumps that are concentrated in these structures to rapidly restore ion gradients following depolarization and neurotransmitter release. Mitochondria may also play important roles in the regulation of synaptic function because of their ability to regulate ROS production and calcium level.

ROS generated in response to synaptic activity are now known to contribute to the regulation of long-term structural and functional changes in neurons [49-52].

Mitochondria have developed the ability of up-taking and releasing calcium. The calcium-handling systems in mitochondria appear to be responsive to various signals and recent findings suggest key role for mitochondria in the regulation of calcium dynamics that control processes such as axon outgrowth and neurotransmitter release [53-55].

The high-energy demands of synapses, together with their high levels of ROS production, renders them at risk during conditions of increased stress, which occur in aging, neurodegenerative disorders and after acute traumatic and ischemic insults.

Energy depletion and/or increased oxidative damage to various synaptic proteins can result in a local dysregulation of calcium homeostasis and synaptic degeneration.

Accordingly, recent studies have shown that dietary and pharmacological interventions that improve energy metabolism efficiency and reduce oxyradical production can prevent synaptic degeneration and neuronal death in experimental models of neurodegenerative disorders [56-61].

CoQ10 supplementation could possibly provide neurons with the energy needed to finalize compensatory neuroplastic changes and in the meanwhile protect synapses from oxidative stress.

Experimental and Clinical Data

CoQ10 exerted neuroprotective effects in several *in vivo* and *in vitro* models.

This molecule proved to be protective against oxidative stress in neuronal cells. Pre-treatment with CoQ10 maintains mitochondrial membrane potential during oxidative stress and reduces the amount of mitochondrial ROS generation [62].

The protective role of CoQ10 was also studied in several toxin models.

Oral administration of CoQ10 exerted significant neuroprotective effects against striatal lesions in rats produced by aminoxyacetic acid and the mitochondrial toxins malonate and 3- NP [63-65].

Oral administration of CoQ10 produced dose-dependent neuroprotective effects against malonate-induced striatal lesions, depletion of ATP, and increases in lactate concentration. Similarly, oral administration of CoQ10 for one week prior to administration of 3-NP resulted in a significant 90% neuroprotection against 3-NP-induced striatal lesions [65].

Coenzyme Q10 effectiveness was evaluated also in cellular and animal models of amyotrophic lateral sclerosis, Parkinson's and Alzheimer's diseases.

CoQ10 was shown to protect against paraquat- and rotenone-induced mitochondrial dysfunction and neuronal cell death in human neuroblastoma (SHSY-5Y) cells and primary rat mesencephalic neurons, respectively [66, 67]. It provided neuroprotection in iron-induced apoptosis in dopaminergic neurons [68].

CoQ10 provided significant protection against MPTP-induced dopamine depletion and loss of TH-IR neurons in aged mice [69].

More recently, dietary administration of CoQ10 resulted in significant protection in a chronic MPTP model induced by the administration of MPTP by Alzet pump for one month [70].

CoQ10 exerted anti-amyloidogenic effects by destabilizing preformed β-amyloid fibrils *in vitro* [71]. Further, CoQ10 protected SHSY5Y neuronal cells from β-amyloid toxicity through inhibition of the MPT pore [72].

CoQ10 treatment decreased brain oxidative stress, Aβ42 levels, β-amyloid plaque area and number, and improved cognitive performance in Tg19959 mice, a transgenic mouse model of AD. High dose CoQ10 significantly extended survival, improved motor performance and grip strength, and reduced brain atrophy in R6/2 HD mice in a dose-dependent manner [73].

CoQ10 produced neuroprotective effects in transgenic mouse models of ALS [74].

Clinical trials testing the neuroprotective activity of CoQ10 in these neurodegenerative diseases have shown promising results [32-38].

Q-TER®: A Water-soluble Formulation of CoQ10

CoQ10 is well known to be a practically insoluble substance, with very poor bioavailability and high stability problems; it is also poorly workable due to its waxylike properties.

Q-TER® is a multicomposite water-soluble formulation of CoQ10, obtained by a patented technology named "terclatration".

This technology consists in a dry grinding process of a ternary mixture constituted by an active substance, a hydrophilic or hydrophobic carrier and a co-grinding auxiliary substance.

The ternary mixture is obtained by mechano-physical activation, a procedure that brings different substances into intimate contact through the administration of energy. This procedure turns a simple mixture of moieties into a multicomposite material (Patent WO/2003/097012).

By definition, in a multicomposite material the chemical moieties of the starting materials are preserved while the physicochemical properties like solubility, stability and dissolution rate are improved.

In particular, Q-TER® consists of a mixture of maltodextrin, acting as a carrier, of CoQ10 molecules (10%w/w), and of sucrester, that serves as bioactivator [75](Figure 2).

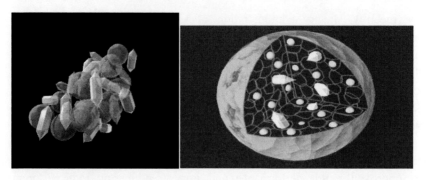

Figure 2. 3-D structure of native CoQ10 (on the left) and of Q-TER® (on the right). In the Q-TER® structure, CoQ10 has been represented in gray, carrier in violet, co-grinder in yellow.

Compared to native CoQ10, the resulting multicomposite is about 200 times more soluble in water while retaining its antioxidant capacity. This allows a greater bioavailability and an improved chemical stability compared to the native form [76].

Q-TER® is manufactured starting from an industrially available native CoQ10 (Kaneka Pharma Europe, Brussels, Belgium).

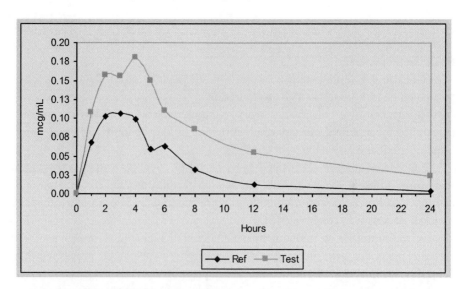

Figure 3. Human plasma levels of Q-TER® (green line) and native CoQ10 (blue line) after single oral administration.

The relative bioavailability of Q-TER® and standard Q10 orally administered to 18 healthy volunteers was evaluated in a single dose, cross-over, randomised, 7 days wash-out study (unpublished data). CoQ10 16 mg, placebo and Q-TER® 160mg were administered to 18 healthy male and female volunteers in fasting condition. Relevant pharmacokinetic parameters ($AUC_{(0-t)}$, $AUC_{(0-24)}$, $AUC_{(0-inf)}$, C_{max}, T_{max} Lz, T ½ and MRT) were evaluated.

The plasma CoQ10 concentrations are represented in Figure 3. The study shows higher bioavailability for the test treatment (Q-TER®) in comparison to the reference one (Standard Q10), when both were administered in fasting conditions.

In a recent study the effectiveness of Q-TER® in preventing noise induced hearing loss was evaluated in a model of acoustic trauma in the guinea pig, in comparison with native CoQ10 [77].

Both treatments were given intraperitoneally 1 h before and once daily for 3 days after pure tone noise exposure (6 kHz for 1 h at 120 dB SPL).

To identify initial signs of apoptosis, scanning electron microscopy for hair cell loss count, active caspase 3 staining and terminal deoxynucleotidyl trasferase mediated dUTP labelling assay were carried out. Besides these morphological studies, functional analysis, such as measuring auditory brainstem responses, were perfomed.

Q-TER® and CoQ10 treatments decreased active caspase 3 expression and the number of apoptotic cells, but animals injected with Q-TER® showed a greater protection from apoptosis and a lower hearing impairment.

These data confirm that solubility of CoQ10 improves the ability of this compound in preventing oxidative injuries that result from mitochondrial dysfunction.

Citicoline

Also known as cytidine 5-diphosphocholine (CDP-choline), citicoline is an essential intermediate in the biosynthetic pathway of structural phospholipids in cell membranes, particularly phosphatidylcholine, via Kennedy pathway.

It is a mononucleotide composed of ribose, cytosine, pyrophosphate, and choline (Figure 4).

Absorption by the oral route is virtually complete, and bioavailability is therefore approximately the same as by the intravenous route. Following administration by oral route, citicoline is rapidly absorbed and then hydrolyzed in the intestinal wall and liver to choline and cytidine, its two main components.

Both metabolites can cross the blood–brain barrier and reach the central nervous system, where they are incorporated into the phospholipid fraction of the cellular membranes.

Acute neuroprotection by citicoline in brain ischemia was first described in experimental studies 3 decades ago [78].

The neuroplasticity enhancing and neurorestorative effects of citicoline have been suggested to be mediated by two leading mechanisms: 1) synthesis of membrane phospholipids, and 2) enhanced production of the neurotransmitter acetylcholine.

Synthesis of Membrane Phospholipids

Phospholipids are the essential constituents of cell membranes and required for maintenance of homeostasis, activity of membrane associated enzymes, coupling of receptor and intracellular signaling, and nerve impulse conduction.

The main phospholipids in humans are phosphatidylcholine, phosphatidylethanolamine, phosphatidylinositol, and sphingomyelin. Formation of citicoline is the rate-limiting step in the formation of phosphatidylcholine through the Kennedy cycle.

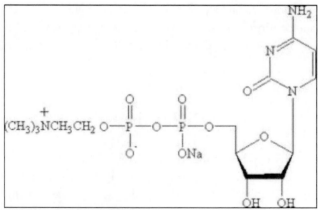

Figure 4. Chemical structure of citicoline.

Cell membrane phospholipids have a very high turnover rate; continuous synthesis of replacement compounds is required to maintain cell integrity in normal circumstances.

Even greater demand of phospholipids' precursors arise in case of cell membrane damage, i.e. lipid peroxidation caused by reactive oxygen species, or to support neurogenesis, axonal sprouting and synaptogenesis.

Exogenously administered citicoline promotes phospholipid synthesis and neural repair.

Animals treated with citicoline in the subacute stroke period showed greater motor recovery and motor neurons structurally were characterized by enhanced dendritic complexity and spine density, suggesting that citicoline therapy supports neuroplastic changes within noninjured regions, mediating functional recovery [79].

Besides supplying cells with choline, citicoline exert anti-apoptotic and anti-necrotic activities, via downregulation of phospholipases [80, 81].

Neurotransmitter Production

Citicoline serves as a choline donor in the biosynthesis of acetylcholine [82]. Acetylcholine is a neurotransmitter that mediates learning and memory and multiple additional nervous system functions, including in auditory pathway.

In animal stroke models, administration of citicoline increases the release of acetylcholine at cholinergic nerve endings and improves attentional, learning, and memory performance.

Besides increasing acetylcholine levels, citicoline supplementation have demonstrated to augment dopamine concentration, likely via enhancing tyrosine hydroxylase activity, inhibiting dopamine reuptake at nerve terminals.

Dopamine is a neurotransmitter involved in movement, attention, and diverse other functions. This neurotransmitter is present also in auditory pathways [83].

Basic Pharmacology and Toxicity

When infused intravenously in humans, citicoline is rapidly hydrolyzed to choline and cytidine, which are delivered to tissues throughout the body.

In healthy volunteers, at the end of a 30-minute infusion, plasma levels of citicoline are already virtually undetectable, whereas choline and cytidine levels are at a peak, with continued elevated circulating concentrations for the following 6 hours.

Delivery by the oral route, though not as rapid as intravenous administration, is virtually complete and bioavailability is therefore approximately the same as by the intravenous route.

Radioactive tracer studies have proved that citicoline efficiently crosses the blood-brain barrier and achieve wide distribution throughout the brain, being incorporated in cortex, white matter, and central gray nuclei.

Exogenous administered citicoline is eventually eliminated very slowly, with small amounts exiting each day by the urinary, fecal, and respiratory routes [83].

Citicoline exhibits a very low toxicity profile [84]. In preclinical studies, a lethal oral dose could not be determined because no deaths occurred at the maximum possible oral dose. No toxic effects were observed in 30-day subacute and 6-month chronic administration toxicity studies of oral citicoline in rodents and dogs. Citicoline supplementation do not cause any changes in blood chemistry, organ histology, or neurological or urinary parameters.

In multiple formal clinical trials with prospective monitoring, no categories of serious adverse events have been reported; uncommon non-serious adverse effects include gastrointestinal distress, restlessness, and irritability, generally within the first few days of treatment.

In a large drug surveillance study analyzing the safety profile of citicoline in 2817 patients, predominantly elderly individuals treated for Alzheimer and vascular dementia, with treatment duration ranging from 2 to 9 weeks, only 5% of patients reported adverse effects; gastrointestinal distress was most common (3.6%), and no patient needed to discontinue therapy due to side effects.

Experimental and Clinical Data

Citicoline have proved its neuroprotective action in several animal models and clinical trials.

Citicoline injected experimentally into the cerebrum of gerbils shortly before artificially-induced ischemia has demonstrated an ability to partially restore phosphatidylcholine levels while inhibiting free fatty acid release, suggesting stabilization of the neuronal membrane [85].

In another gerbil study, citicoline restored ischemia-depleted levels of phosphatidylcholine, sphingomyelin, and cardiolipin after one day of reperfusion. In addition, this study found that after three days of reperfusion, citicoline increased both glutathione levels and glutathione reductase activity, suggesting citicoline may contribute to reduction of oxidative stress [86].

In another study, citicoline was tested in an animal stroke model. Temporary focal ischemia was artificially induced in rats via blockage of the right middle cerebral artery and maintained for two hours. In the rats administered 500 mg/kg of citicoline for the next 6 days, the "infarct volumes" (volume of damaged brain tissue at ischemia sites) and brain edema were significantly smaller than in the placebo group [87].

A total of 13 randomized clinical trials of citicoline in acute and subacute stroke have been reported in the literature [82]. The European clinical trials showed that citicoline improved global and neurological function and promoted earlier motor and cognitive recovery.

A large multi-center study in Japan found that CDP-choline showed improvement in a global outcome rating scale. Four major clinical trials in the USA have provided ambiguous results, and thus the beneficial effects of CDP-choline have not been established.

The European and Japanese trials used i.v. administration in contrast to oral route used in the USA trials.

As loss of neuronal and glial membrane integrity is a final common pathway of cell injury arising from many disease processes, citicoline has been tested in a wide variety of neurologic conditions aside from focal stroke.

Most directly relevant to stroke are studies in patients with late-life cognitive impairment that have preponderantly targeted patients with vascular cognitive impairment or mixed vascular and Alzheimer disease.

The most recent Cochrane review of these studies identified 14 trials enrolling a total of 1051 patients and concluded that there was some evidence of a positive effect upon memory, behavior, and global functioning, though not on attention [88].

Since citicoline increases dopamine production in the striatum and has shown benefits in a variety of experimental models of Parkinson disease, several small open-label and controlled clinical trials performed in the 1970s and 1980s have been performed and results suggested potential benefits of citicoline in Parkinson patients [83].

Glaucoma may in part be mediated by ischemic injury to retinal and postretinal structures due to elevated ocular tension. Small controlled trials using visual electrophysiologic endpoints have suggested a beneficial effect of citicoline. Nonarteritic ischemic optic neuropathy is a chronic, small artery–mediated ischemic injury to the intraocular optic nerve. A recent randomized but open-label trial in 26 patients found improved visual acuity and visual evoked potentials in citicoline treated patients when compared with control subjects [89].

Conclusion

Among potential molecules enhancing neuroplasticity, CoQ10 and citicoline are promising and characterized by an excellent safety profile.

These two compounds benefit from complementary activities within the cells, in terms of protection from intrinsic apoptosis pathway start and of support of structural and neurochemical changes involving synapses.

CoQ10, thanks to its strong direct and indirect antioxidant activity and its close proximity to membrane unsaturated lipids, can prevent lipid peroxidation caused by reactive oxygen species.

Citicoline can intervene in case of membrane damages, supplying the cells with phospholipids' precursors.

Great demand for phospholipid generation arises to support neurogenesis, axonal sprouting, and synaptogenesis. Since formation of citicoline is the rate-limiting step in the synthesis of phosphatidylcholine, exogenously administered citicoline accelerates phospholipid synthesis and neural repair. Moreover plastic changes of neural networks require huge amount of energy, since they involve the outgrowth of axons and the active transport of various molecules from the cell body to the synapse. CoQ10 supplementation sustains mitochondrial oxidative metabolism, directly implicated in synaptic remodelling.

Citicoline serves as a choline donor in the biosynthesis of acetylcholine.

Exogenously administered citicoline increases acetylcholine synthesis, by providing choline, and dopamine concentration at synaptic cleft, likely via enhancing tyrosine hydroxylase activity, inhibiting dopamine reuptake at nerve terminals.

CoQ10 bioenergetic activity aids to supply neurons with ATP amount needed for neurotransmitters synthesis.

Scientific evidences about citicoline and CoQ10 neuroprotective and neurorepairing activities, gathered in several models of neurodegeneration and acute neuronal damage, suggest great potential of these active principles in enhancing and directing neuroplastic changes of central auditory pathway after a peripheral damage.

Even if clinical data in audiological field are limited, these assumptions lay the foundations for rational use of these compounds in hearing loss and tinnitus prevention.

Citicoline and Q-TER® (water soluble CoQ10) are included in a nutraceutical product named Acuval®, together with other otoprotective compounds, such as

Gingko biloba (in the form of phytosome), L-arginine, vitamins A, E, B1, B2, B6, B12, magnesium, selenium and zinc.

References

[1]   Bhagavan HN, Chopra RK. Coenzyme Q10: Absorption, tissue uptake, metabolism and pharmacokinetics. *Free Radical Research,* 2006, Vol. 40, 5: 445-453

[2]   Ernster L, Dallner G. Biochemical, physiological and medical aspects of ubiquinone function. *Biochim Biophys Acta,* 1995, 1271:195–204.

[3]   Zhang Y, Turunen M, Appelkvist EL. Restricted uptake of dietary coenzyme Q is in contrast to the unrestricted uptake of a-tocopherol into rat organs and cells. *J Nutr,* 1996, 126:2089–2097.

[4]   Lenaz G, Fato R, Formiggini G, Genova ML. The role of Coenzyme Q in mitochondrial electron transport. *Mitochondrion* 2007, S7, S8–33.

[5]   Yu CA, Zhang KP, Deng H, Xia D, Klm H, Deisenhofer J, Yu L. Structure and reaction mechanisms of the multifunctional mitochondrial cytochrome bc1 complex. *Biofactors* 1999, 9:103–110.

[6]   Takahashi T, Okamoto T, Mori K, Sayo H, Kishi T. Distribution of ubiquinone and ubiquinol homologues in rat tissues and subcellular fraction. *Lipids* 1993, 28:803–809.

[7]   Quinn PJ, Fabisiak JP, Kagan VE. Expansion of the antioxidant function of vitamin E by coenzyme Q. *Biofactors* 1999, 9:149–154.

[8]   Zhang Y, Aberg F, Appelkvist EL, Dallner G, Ernster L. Uptake of dietary coenzyme Q supplement is limited in rats. *J Nutr* 1995, 125:446–453.

[9]   Chopra RK, Goldman R, Sinatra ST, Bhagavan HN. Relative bioavailability of coenzyme Q10 formulations in human subjects. *Int J Vitam Nutr Res* 1998, 68:109–113.

[10] Miles MV, Horn P, Miles L, Tang P, Steele P, DeGrauw T. Bioequivalence of coenzyme Q10 from over-the-counter supplements. *Nutr Res* 2002, 22:919–929.

[11] Zaghloul AA, Gurley B, Khan M, Bhagavan H, Chopra R, Reddy I. Bioavailability assessment of oral coenzyme Q10 formulations in dogs. *Drug Dev Ind Pharm,* 2002, 28:1195–1200

[12] Katayama K, Fujita T. Studies on the lymphatic absorption of 10,20-(3H)-coenzyme Q10 in rats. *Chem Pharm Bull,* 1972, 250:2585–2592.

[13] Craft NE, Tucker RT, Chitchumroonchokchai C, Failla M, Bhagavan HN.
      Assessment of coenzyme Q10 bioavailability using a coupled in vitro
      digestion/Caco-2 human intestinal cellmodel. *FASEB J*, 2005,19:A449.

[14] Elmberger PG, Kalen A, Brunk UT, Dallner G. Discharge of newly-
      synthesized dolichol and ubiquinone with lipoproteins to rat liver perfusate
      and to the bile. *Lipids,* 1989, 24:919–930.

[15] Traber MG, Lne JC, Lagmay NR, Kayden HJ. Studies on the transfer of
      tocopherol between lipoproteins. *Lipids,* 1992, 27:657–663.

[16] Laaksonen R, Riihimaki A, Laitila J, Martensson K, Tikkanen MJ, Himberg
      JJ. Serum and muscle tissue ubiquinone levels in healthy subjects. *J Lab
      Clin Med,* 1995, 125:517–521.

[17] Aberg F, Appelkvist EL, Dallner G, Ernster L. Distribution and redox state
      of ubiquinones in rat and human tissues. *Arch Biochem Biophys*, 1992,
      295:230–234.

[18] Miles MV, Horn PS, Morrison JA, Tang PH, DeGrauw T, Pesce AJ. Plasma
      coenzyme Q10 reference intervals, but not redox status, are affected by
      gender and race in self-reported healthy adults. *Clin Chim Acta*, 2003,
      332:123–132.

[19] Lonnrot K, Metsa-Katela T, Molnar G, Ahonen J-P, Latvala M, Peltola J,
      Pietila T, Alho H. The effect of acsorbate and ubiquinone supplementation
      on plasma and CSF total antioxidant capacity. *Free Rad Biol Med,* 1996,
      21:211–217.

[20] Langsjoen PH, Langsjoen PH, Folkers K. Long-term efficacy and safety of
      coenzyme Q10 therapy for idiopathic dilated cardiomyopathy. *Am J
      Cardiol,* 1990, 65:421–423.

[21] Jones K, Hughes K, Mischley L, McKenna D. Coenzyme Q10: Efficacy,
      safety, and use. Int *J Integr Med,* 2002, 4:28–43.

[22] Williams KD, Maneke JD, Abdelhameed M, Hall RL, Palmer TE, Kitano
      M, Hidaka T. Week oral gavage chronic toxicity study with ubiquinone in
      rats with a 4-week recovery. *J Agric Food Chem*, 1999, 47:3756–3763.

[23] Kieburtz K (The Huntington Study Group). A randomized placebo-
      controlled trial of coenzyme Q10 and remacemide in Huntington's disease.
      Neurology, 2001, 57:397–404.

[24] Shultz CW, Oakes D, Kieburtz K, Beal FL, Haas R, Plumb S, Juncos JL,
      Nutt J, Shoulson I, Carter J, Kompoliti K, Perlmutter JS, Reich S, Stern M,
      Watts RL, Kurlan R, Molho E, Harrison M, Lew M. and the Parkinson
      Study Group. Effects of coenzyme Q10 in early Parkinson disease. *Arch
      Neurol,* 2002, 59:1541–1550.

[25] Shults CW, Beal MF, Song D, Fontaine D. Pilot trial of high dosages of
       coenzyme Q10 in patients with Parkinson's disease. *Exp Neurol,* 2004,
       188:491–494.
[26] Ferrante KL, Shefner J, Zhang H, Betensky R, O'Brien M, Yu H, Fantasia
       M, Taft J, Beal MF, Traynor B, Newhall K, Donofrio P, Caress J, Ashburn
       C, Freiburg B, O'Neill C, Paladenech C, Walker T, Pestronk A, Abrams B,
       Florence J, Renna R, Schierbecker J, Malkus B, Cudkowicz M. Tolerance
       of high-dose (3000 mg/day) Coenzyme Q10 in ALS. *Neurology,* 2005,
       65:1834–1836.
[27] Le Prell CG, Hughes LF, Miller JM. Free radical scavengers vitamins A, C,
       and E plus magnesium reduce noisetrauma. *Free Radic. Biol. Med.* 2007,
       42, 1454–1463.
[28] Henderson D, Bielefeld EC, Harris KC, Hu BH. The role of oxidative stress
       in noise-induced hearing loss. *Ear Hear,* 2006, 27, 1–19.
[29] Green DR, Reed JC. Mitochondria and apoptosis. *Science,*1998, 281:1309–
       1312.
[30] Van De Water TR, Lallemend F, Eshraghi AA, Ahsan S, He J, Guzman J,
       Polak M, Malgrange B, Lefebvre PP, Staecker H, Balkany TJ. Caspases, the
       enemy within, and their role in oxidative stress-induced apoptosis of inner
       ear sensory cells. *Otol. Neurol,* 2004, 25: 627–632.
[31] Reed JC. Mechanisms of apoptosis. *Am. J. Pathol.,* 2000,157:1415–1430.
[32] Storch A, Jost WH, Vieregge P, Spiegel J, Greulich W, Durner J, Müller T,
       Kupsch A, Henningsen H, Oertel WH, Fuchs G, Kuhn W, Niklowitz P,
       Koch R, Herting B, Reichmann H; German Coenzyme Q(10) Study Group.
       Randomized, double-blind, placebo-controlled trial on symptomatic effects
       of coenzyme Q(10) in Parkinson disease. *Arch Neurol.,* 2007, 64(7):938-44.
[33] Shults CW, Flint Beal M, Song D, Fontaine D. Pilot trial of high dosages of
       coenzyme Q10 in patients with Parkinson's disease. *Exp Neurol.,*
       2004,188(2):491-4.
[34] Shults CW, Oakes D, Kieburtz K, Beal MF, Haas R, Plumb S, Juncos JL,
       Nutt J, Shoulson I, Carter J, Kompoliti K, Perlmutter JS, Reich S, Stern M,
       Watts RL, Kurlan R, Molho E, Harrison M, Lew M; Parkinson Study
       Group. Effects of coenzyme Q10 in early Parkinson disease: evidence of
       slowing of the functional decline. *Arch Neurol.,* 2002, 59(10):1541-50.
[35] Strijks E, Kremer HP, Horstink MW. Q10 therapy in patients with
       idiopathic Parkinson's disease. *Mol Aspects Med.,* 1997, 18 Suppl:S237-40.
[36] Huntington Study Group A randomized, placebo-controlled trial of
       coenzyme Q10 and remacemide in Huntington's disease. *Neurology,*
       2001,14, 57(3):397-404.

[37] Levy G, Kaufmann P, Buchsbaum R, Montes J, Barsdorf A, Arbing R, Battista V, Zhou X, Mitsumoto H, Levin B, Thompson JL. A two-stage design for a phase II clinical trial of coenzyme Q10 in ALS. *Neurology*, 2006, 14;66(5):660-3.

[38] Ferrante KL, Shefner J, Zhang H, Betensky R, O'Brien M, Yu H, Fantasia M, Taft J, Beal MF, Traynor B, Newhall K, Donofrio P, Caress J, Ashburn C, Freiberg B, O'Neill C, Paladenech C, Walker T, Pestronk A, Abrams B, Florence J, Renna R, Schierbecker J, Malkus B, Cudkowicz M. Tolerance of high-dose (3,000 mg/day) coenzyme Q10 in ALS. *Neurology*, 2005, 13;65(11):1834-6.

[39] Naderi J et al. Water-soluble formulation of Coenzyme Q10 inhibits Bax-induced destabilization of mitochondria in mammalian cells. *Apoptosis*, 2006, 11: 1359–1369.

[40] Papucci L. et al. Coenzyme q10 prevents apoptosis by inhibiting mitochondrial depolarization independently of its free radical scavenging property. *J. Biol. Chem.* , 2003, 278: 28220–28228.

[41] Beal MF. Bioenergetic approaches for neuroprotection in Parkinson's disease. *Ann. Neurol,* 2003, 53(Suppl 3): S39–47.

[42] Beal MF. Therapeutic effects of coenzyme Q10 in neurodegenerative diseases. *Methods Enzymol.,* 2004, 382: 473–487.

[43] Pfister KK Cytoplasmic dynein and microtubule transport in the axon: the action connection. *Mol. Neurobiol.*, 1999, 20:81–91.

[44] Pollard TD, Blanchoin L, Mullins RD Molecular mechanisms controlling actin filament dynamics in nonmuscle cells. *Annu. Rev. Biophys. Biomol. Struct.*, 2000, 29:545–576.

[45] Pantaloni D, Le Clainche C, Carlier MF. Mechanism of actin-based motility. *Science*, 2001, 292: 1502–1506.

[46] Farrell CM, Mackey AT, Klumpp LM, Gilbert SP. The role of ATP hydrolysis for kinesin processivity. *J. Biol. Chem.* 2002, 277, 17,079–17,087.

[47] Hollenbeck PJ. The pattern and mechanism of mitochondrial transport in axons. *Front. Biosci.,* 1996, 1:d91–d102.

[48] Dedov VN, Armati PJ, Roufogalis BD. Three-dimensional organisation of mitochondrial clusters in regenerating dorsal root ganglion (DRG) neurons from neonatal rats: evidence for mobile mitochondrial pools. *J. Peripher. Nerv. Syst.*, 2000, 5: 3–10.

[49] Knapp LT, Klann E. Potentiation of hippocampal synaptic transmission by superoxide requires the oxidative activation of protein kinase C. *J. Neurosci.*, 2002, 22: 674–683.

[50] Thiels E, Urban NN, Gonzalez-Burgos GR, Kanterewicz BI, Barrionuevo G, Chu CT et al. Impairment of long-term potentiation and associative memory in mice that overexpress extracellular superoxide dismutase. *J. Neurosci.*, 2000, 20: 7631–7639.

[51] Colton CA, Fagni L, Gilbert D. The action of hydrogen peroxide on paired pulse and longterm potentiation in the hippocampus. *Free Radic. Biol. Med.*, 1989, 7: 3–8.

[52] Auerbach JM, Segal M. Peroxide modulation of slow onset potentiation in rat hippocampus. *J. Neurosci.*, 1997, 17: 8695–8701.

[53] Boitier E, Rea R, Duchen MR. Mitochondria exert a negative feedback on the propagation of intracellular Ca2+ waves in rat cortical astrocytes. *J. Cell Biol.*, 1999, 145: 795–808.

[54] Mattson MP, Partin J. Evidence for mitochondrial control of neuronal polarity. *J. Neurosci. Res.*, 1999, 56: 8–20.

[55] Bootman MD, Lipp P, Berridge MJ. The organisation and functions of local Ca(2+) signals. *J. Cell Sci.*, 2001, 114: 2213–2222.

[56] Persky AM, Brazeau GA. Clinical pharmacology of the dietary supplement creatine monohydrate. *Pharmacol. Rev.*, 2001, 53: 161–176.

[57] Sullivan PG, Geiger JD, Mattson MP, Scheff SW. Dietary supplement creatine protects against traumatic brain injury. *Ann. Neurol.*, 2000, 48: 723–729.

[58] Tarnopolsky MA, Beal MF. Potential for creatine and other therapies targeting cellular energy dysfunction in neurological disorders. *Ann. Neurol.*, 2001, 49: 561–574.

[59] Mark RJ, Hensley K, Butterfield DA, Mattson MP. Amyloid beta-peptide impairs ion motive ATPase activities: evidence for a role in loss of neuronal Ca2+ homeostasis and cell death. *J. Neurosci.*, 1995, 15: 6239–6249.

[60] Gurney ME, Pu H, Chiu AY, Dal Canto MC, Polchow CY, Alexander DD, et al. Motor neuron degeneration in mice that express a human Cu,Zn superoxide dismutase mutation. *Science*, 1994, 264: 1772–1775.

[61] Kitagawa K, Matsumoto M, Kuwabara K, Takasawa K, Tanaka S, Sasaki T, et al. Protective effect of apolipoprotein E against ischemic neuronal injury is mediated through antioxidant action. *J. Neurosci. Res.*, 2002, 68: 226–232.

[62] Somayajulu M et al. Role of mitochondria in neuronal cell death induced by oxidative stress; neuroprtection by Coenzyme Q10. *Neurobiol. Dis.*, 2005, 18: 618–627.

[63] Beal MF et al. Coenzyme Q10 and nicotinammide block striatal lesions produced by the mitochondrial toxin malonate. *Ann. Neurol.*, 1994, 36: 882–888.

[64] Brouillet E. et al. Aminooxyacetic acid striatal lesions attenuated by 1,3-butanediol and coenzyme Q10. *Neurosci. Lett.*, 1994, 177: 58–62.

[65] Matthews RT et al. Coenzyme Q10 administration increases brain mitochondrial concentrations and exerts neuroprotective effects. *Proc. Natl. Acad. Sci. USA,* 1998, 95: 8892–8897.

[66] McCarthy S et al. Paraquat induces oxidative stress and neuronal cell death; neuroprotection by water-soluble Coenzyme Q10. *Toxicol. Appl. Pharmacol.*, 2004, 201: 21–31.

[67] Moon Y et al. 2005. Mitochondrial membrane depolarization and the selective death of dopaminergic neurons by rotenone: protective effect of coenzyme Q10. *J. Neurochem.* 93: 1199–1208.

[68] Kooncumchoo P et al. Coenzyme Q(10) provides neuroprotection in iron-induced apoptosis in dopaminergic neurons. *J. Mol. Neurosci.*, 2006, 28: 125–141.

[69] Beal MF et al. Coenzyme Q10 attenuates the 1-methyl-4-phenyl-1,2,3,tetrahydropyridine (MPTP) induced loss of striatal dopamine and dopaminergic axons in aged mice. *Brain Res,* 1998, 783: 109–114.

[70] Cleren C et al. Therapeutic effects of coenzyme Q10 (CoQ10) and reduced CoQ10 in the MPTP model of parkinsonism. *J Neurochem.*, 2008, 104(6):1613-21.

[71] Ono K et al. Preformed beta-amyloid fibrils are destabilized by coenzyme Q10 in vitro. *Biochem. Biophys. Res. Commun.*, 2005, 330: 111–116.

[72] Li G. et al. Coenzyme Q10 protects SHSY5Y neuronal cells from beta amyloid toxicity and oxygen-glucose deprivation by inhibiting the opening of the mitochondrial permeability transition pore. *Biofactors*, 2005, 25: 97–107.

[73] Ferrante RJ et al. Therapeutic effects of coenzyme Q10 and remacemide in transgenic mouse models of Huntington's disease. *J. Neurosci.* 2002, 22: 1592–1599.

[74] Matthews RT et al. Coenzyme Q10 administration increases brain mitochondrial concentrations and exerts neuroprotective effects. *Proc. Natl. Acad. Sci. USA* 1998. 95: 8892–8897.

[75] Corvi Mora P, Canal T, Fortuna F, Ruzzier F. An Innovative Technology For Improving Solubility And Antioxidant Properties Of Coenzyme Q10. *Oxygen Society Of California Congress "Oxidants And Antioxidants In Biology"*, Alba 7–10 September 2005..

[76] Corvi Mora P, Canal T, Fortuna F, Ruzzier F. Composition containing micronutrients with improved anti-oxidant activity and use thereof. WO/2007/009997 (2007).

[77] Fetoni AR, Piacentini R, Fiorita A, Paludetti G, Troiani D. Water-soluble Coenzyme Q10 formulation (Q-ter) promotes outer hair cell survival in a guinea pig model of noise induced hearing loss (NIHL). *Brain Res.*, 2009,1257:108-16.

[78] Boismare F, Le Poncin M, Lefrancois J, Lecordier JC. Action of cytidine diphosphocholine on functional and hemodynamic effects of cerebral ischemia in cats. *Pharmacology,* 1978, 17: 15-20.

[79] Hurtado O, Cardenas A, Pradillo JM, et al. A chronic treatment with CDP-choline improves functional recovery and increases neuronal plasticity after experimental stroke. *Neurobiol Dis.*, 2007, 26:105-111.

[80] Krupinski J, Ferrer I, Barrachina M, et al. CDPcholine reduces pro-caspase and cleaved caspase- caspase- 3 expression, nuclear DNA fragmentation, and specific PARP-cleaved products of caspase activation following middle cerebral artery occlusion in the rat. *Neuropharmacology,* 2002, 42: 846-854.

[81] Adibhatla RM, Hatcher JF, Larsen EC, et al. CDP-choline significantly restores phosphatidylcholine levels by differentially affecting phospholipase A2 and CTP: phosphocholine cytidylyltransferase after stroke. *J Biol Chem.*, 2006, 281:6718-6725.

[82] Adibhatla RM, Hatcher JF, Dempsey RJ. Citicoline: Neuroprotective mechanisms in cerebral ischemia. *J Neurochem,* 2002, 80:12–23.

[83] Saver JL. Citicoline: Update on a Promising and Widely Available Agent for Neuroprotection and Neurorepair *REVIEWS IN NEUROLOGICAL DISEASES,* 2008, VOL. 5 NO. 4

[84] Secades JJ, Lorenzo JL. Citicoline: pharmacological and clinical review, 2006 update. *Methods Find Exp Clin Pharmacol.*, 2006;28 (suppl B):1-56.

[85] Rao AM, Hatcher JF, Dempsey RJ. CDP-choline: neuroprotection in transient forebrain ischemia of gerbils. *J Neurosci Res.,* 1999, 1;58(5):697-705.

[86] Adibhatla RM, Hatcher JF, Dempsey RJ. Effects of citicoline on phospholipid and glutathione levels in transient cerebral ischemia. *Stroke,* 2001,32(10):2376-81.

[87] Ataus SA, Onal MZ, Ozdem SS, et al. The effects of citicoline and lamotrigine alone and in combination following permanent middle cerebral artery occlusion in rats. *Int J Neurosci.* 2004, 114:183-196.

[88] Fioravanti M, Yanagi M. Cytidinediphosphocholine (CDP-choline) for cognitive and behavioural disturbances associated with chronic cerebral disorders in the elderly. *Cochrane Database Syst Rev*. 2005:CD000269.
[89] Parisi V, Coppola G, Ziccardi L, et al. Cytidine-5-diphosphocholine (Citicoline): a pilotstudy in patients with non-arteritic ischaemicoptic neuropathy. *Eur J Neurol.*, 2008, 15:465-474.

In: Neuroplasticity in the Auditory Brainstem   ISBN 978-1-61761-949-6
Editor: Angelo Salami, pp. 119-141   © 2011 Nova Science Publishers, Inc.

Chapter VIII

New Drugs to Improve the Neuroplasticity of the Central Auditory Pathway

**A. Salami, R. Mora, M. Dellepiane,
V. Santomauro, and L. Guastini**
ENT Department, University of Genoa, Italy

Abstract

Neuroplasticity is classically accepted as the capacity of neurons to change the shape of their connection tree. This ability is made possible by messenger pathways that mediate signal transduction in the brain. The short- and long-term modulatory effects that neurotransmitters exert on their target neurons via regulation of intracellular messenger pathways can be viewed as the basis of neural plasticity.

Besides the brain's intracellular messenger pathways are themselves targets of long-term regulation and contribute prominently to drug-induced neural plasticity.

There are three general types of mechanisms by which a drug could alter levels of a protein: regulation of gene transcription, regulation of RNA translation and turnover, or regulation of protein turnover. Studies of drug regulation of gene expression to date have focused almost exclusively on two families of transcription factors: CREB (cAMP response element binding protein) and related proteins mediate many of the effects of cAMP and probably Ca^{2+} on gene expression. CREB's transcriptional activity is regulated primarily via its phosphorylation by cAMP-dependent and Ca^{2+}-dependent protein kinases. Increasing evidence demonstrates that psychotropic drug treatments can regulate CREB function in the brain, presumably by influencing these intracellular pathways.

c-Fos, c-Jun, and products of related immediate early genes (IEGs) are regulated in the brain by diverse types of stimuli, including numerous drug and other treatments. Extracellular stimuli are thought to regulate these transcription factors primarily by regulating their expression, possibly mediated via the cAMP- or Ca^{2+}-dependent phosphorylation of CREB or CREB-like proteins. However, Fos- and Jun-like proteins are also known to be phosphorylated by many protein kinases, and this serves to further regulate their transcriptional activity.

On the basis of these studies is evident that neuroplasticity may be present even in the elderly. In order to evaluate the neuroplasticity in older people, the purpose of this chapter was to study the effects of an antioxidant agent (Q-TER®) in the treatment of presbyacusis.

Introduction

The last 20 years of research has made it clear that some drugs produce several changes in brain function, caused by repeated pharmacological insult to the brain circuits that regulate how a person interprets and behaviorally responds to motivationally relevant stimuli. Thus, some drugs strongly interact with and change the brain circuits that permit us to learn about and behaviorally adapt to important environmental stimuli, whether it be how to best approach rewards such as food or sex, or to avoid dangerous situations [1].

By changing motivational circuitry, addictive drugs impair the development of behavioral strategies towards biological stimuli in favor of progressively greater orientation of behavior towards drug-seeking and drug-taking strategies [2,3]. Importantly, these changes are long-lasting and, at present, not readily reversed [2,3].

These changes in brain function are called with the term of neuroplasticity. Neuroplasticity (brain plasticity or cortical plasticity) refers to the modifications that occur in the organization of the brain, and in particular changes that occur to the location of specific information processing functions, as a results of acquired brain injury.

Neuroplasticity allows the neurons to compensate for injury and disease and to adjust their activities in response to new situations or to changes in their environment.

Neuroplasticity is classically accepted as the capacity of neurons to change the shape of their connection tree. Neuroplasticity appears during development and maturation of both central and peripheral nervous systems. It can also, as a reactive process, be observed after nerve lesion. Neuroplasticity is involved in higher brain functions, as learning, memory or language. These processes are mainly conducted by trophic factors and by neurotransmitters, in particular NMDA receptor (N-methyl-D-aspartate) and GABA (γ-aminobutyric acid) that participate in shape changes and functional adaptation of neurons. Glutamate is a major transmitter in central pain pathways. The excitatory effect of glutamate is mediated by two main types of ionotropic receptors: NMDA and AMPA (named after the selective agonist α-amino-3-hydroxy-5-methyl-isoxasole-4-propionic acid). The NMDA receptors contribute to normal excitatory transmission and have special functions related to synaptic plasticity [4,5].

There are different degrease of plasticity on brain system [4,5]:

a) some systems appear strongly determined and change very little even under extreme alterations of experience, e.g., complete deafness or blindness;

b) other neural systems do change considerably when experience is different but only during certain, limited "sensitive" time periods and these time differ for different system;

c) a third of neural systems appear modifiable by experience throughout life.

Neuroplasticity, caused by drugs, can be divided into two categories [1]:

• first, relatively transient changes in neuronal function that continue for hours up to weeks of drug abstinence (*transient neuroplasticity*);

• relatively stable changes lasting from weeks to being relatively permanent changes (*permanent neuroplasticity*).

Transient neuroplasticity corresponds to the necessary changes that are antecedent to developing a new activity, whereas stable neuroplasticity corresponds to the stable information that is retrieved to guide the execution of learned activity. The development of permanent neuroplasticity is typically achieved through repeated use of the drug, and involves many relatively short-lived changes in brain chemistry and physiology based largely on the molecular pharmacology of the drug itself [6].

The permanent neuroplasticity is based on enduring changes in the synaptic physiology of brain circuits responding to important environmental stimuli, as drugs administrations.

There have been large advances over the last decade in our understanding of the underlying brain circuitry and neurotransmitters playing key roles in how memory is acquired, and the learned behaviors executed [7].

The following three phases of neuroplasticity can be inferred using drug sel-administration protocols [8]:

- the acquisition of drug self-administration represents acute neuroplasticity;
- patterns of daily self-administration represent neuroplasticity associated with the habitual drug use;
- the reinstatement of drug seeking represents neuroplasticity underlying relapse.

The cellular responses to acute drug administration are generally short lived, are closely to the molecular site of drug action and are similar to plasticity identified in vitro models of synaptic plasticity, including the induction of immediate early gene (IEG) products such as c-Fos, Homer 1a, NAC-1 and Narp. Unfortunately, it is unclear which of these changes are antecedents to habitual drug use because they have not been validated in animal models of the acquisition of drug self-administration [8]. However, a few IEGs induced by psycho stimulant administration have been linked to behavioral plasticity in which repeated no contingent psycho stimulant administration produces a progressive increase in locomotor activity [8].

The second temporal category of drug-induced neuroplasticity mediates habitual drug use and is characterized by changes in proteins that emerge with repeated drug exposure and then disappear during withdrawal. Included in this category are transcription factors such as proteins regulating dopamine and glutamate transmission [8].

The form of drug-induced neuroplasticity that has been most successfully evaluated in animal models endures for weeks of drug abstinence and may underlie relapse. Moreover the validation between drug-induced neuroplasticity and the reinstatement model of relapse has led to identification of new pharmacotherapeutic targets such as the cysteine-glutamate exchanger and glutamate receptor subtypes [8].

Attempts to link molecular neuroplasticity with the physiology of neuronal networks have been another important outcome of integrating enduring drug-induced neuroplasticity with the reinstatement model.

Presbyacusis is defined as a progressive bilateral symmetrical age related sensorineural hearing loss. The hearing loss is confined to higher frequencies (in the early stages).

Presbyacusis is an added problem for the elderly who have a tendency to compensate for their loss of vision through their intact sense of hearing. They even tend to get isolated and become a social recluse due to this problem.

In order to evaluate the the neuroplasticity in older people, the purpose of this chapter was to evaluate the effects of an atioxidant agent (Q-TER®) in the treatment of presbyacusis.

Antioxidant Agents

The antioxidant agent can stimulate neuroplasticity mechanisms and have a neuroprotection action. Neuroprotection represents the totality of mechanisms and strategies used to increase the nervous cell's resistance to damaging agents. The objective of neuroprotection is represented by the limitation of neuronal dysfunction/death due to different aggressions on the central nervous system and the struggle to maintain the integrity of the cellular interactions as high as possible so that the nervous functions should be conserved [9].

The strategy of the antioxidant treatment consists in interfering with the molecular cascades that determine first neuronal dysfunction and then neuronal death. Several etiological agents or biological processes may trigger the same molecular cascades which will finally lead to neuronal death [9].

There are two main biological models of cellular death. The first is the necrosis during which a failure of cellular homeostasis installs after certain types of aggression (mechanic, anoxic, etc.). It is the result of the extracellular environment alterations occurred with such intensity that the cell's homeostatic system isn't anymore able to compensate them. The cell becomes excessively permeable and the content is eliminated into the extracellular space [10].

The second type of cellular death is called apoptosis and is an active suicide process during which the cell is using its own mechanisms to initiate a series of events leading to digestion of several cellular components. During necrosis the edema causes osmotic lysis, the cell dying passively. In the extracellular environment are liberated products that will initiate the inflammation [11].

Apoptosis is an active process, strictly controlled genetically, necessitating ATP. The cell is preparing itself, the final result consisting of apoptotic bodies. The apoptotic cell death doesn't trigger inflammation. The last tendencies of the scientific world reserves the term "apoptosis" for the physiological process that helps the normal, healthy organism to control the number and quality of its cells. The programmed cellular death processes that occur in pathological situations – from degenerescence to citotoxicity – are called "apoptotic-like" processes. These entities form in fact the target for the citoprotective therapy, a therapy gaining more and more popularity with the clarification of the intimate pathophysiology of many diseases that evolve with cellular loss [11].

Both enzymatic and non-enzymatic defense mechanisms are present in the cell to protect its integrity and functions. The components of these defense systems can be divided into two main groups [12]:

- antioxidant enzymes including superoxide dismutase (SOD), catalase (CAT) and glutathione peroxidase (GSH-Px);
- small endogenous antioxidant molecules such as glutathione (GSH), coenzyme Q (CoQ) and urate.

Other exogenous antioxidants, such as tocopherols (vitamin E), ascorbate (vitamin C), vitamin A and carotenoids and some metals, essential for the function of antioxidant enzymes, are of dietary origin [13].

CoQ or ubiquinone is a redox-active and lipophilic substance present in most cellular membranes. It consists of a quinone head attached to a chain of isoprene units numbering 9 or 10 (CoQ9 or CoQ10) in different mammal species. CoQ10 has a fundamental role in cellular bioenergetics as a cofactor in the mitochondrial electron transport chain (respiratory chain) and is therefore essential for the production of ATP [14]. CoQ10 functions as a mobile redox agent shuttling electrons and protons in the electron transport chain. CoQ is highly efficient in preventing lipid, protein and DNA oxidation and it is continuously regenerated by intracellular reduction systems [14,15].

CoQ10 in its reduced form as the hydroquinone (ubiquinol) is a potent lipophilic antioxidant and is capable of recycling and regenerating other antioxidants such as tocopherol and ascorbate [15]. In some pathologic processes when tissue CoQ content is decreased it may be advantageous to supplement CoQ by dietary administration [15].

CoQ10 is a mobile electron carrier in the mitochondria and is one of the two endogenous antioxidants that delay or prevent oxidation of membrane-bound lipid peroxide free radicals. It is clinically used and tried for treatment of cardiac, neurologic, oncologic and immunologic disorders [16-18].

Vitamin E (Vit E) is a family of lipid-soluble vitamins, of which -tocopherol is the most potent. Vit E has been found to act as an antioxidant in cells, interrupting the propagation of lipid peroxidation in the plasma membrane, preserving membrane integrity [19]. Thus, a number of studies have been carried out to determine the protective effects of Vit E in different biological models of injury [19]. Similarly, a joint action of both CoQ and Vit E against cellular oxidative damage has also been proposed. CoQ has been demonstrated to serve the dual functions of an electron carrier/proton translocator in the respiratory chain and an antioxidant by directly scavenging radicals or indirectly by regenerating Vit E [19].

Q-TER® is a multicomposite water-soluble formulation of CoQ10, obtained by a patented technology named "terclatration". In particular, Q-TER® consists of a mixture of maltodextrin, acting as a carrier, of CoQ10 molecules (10%w/w), and of sucrester, that serves as bioactivator [20].

Compared to native CoQ10, the resulting multicomposite is about 200 times more soluble in water: this allows a greater bioavailability and an improved chemical stability compared to native form [21]. Q-TER® is manufactured using an industrially available native CoQ10 (Kaneka Pharma Europe, Brussels, Belgium).

Methods

The study was conducted according to the Revised Declaration of Helsinki and The Good Clinical Practice Guidelines. All procedures were carried out in accordance with the local ethics committee's protocol.

A total of 66 patients aged between 56 and 74 years (69 years old on average) with presbyacusis were included and completed the trial, between September 2008 and November 2009, among 120 patients eligible during the study period. The patients were equally divided, at random, into three numerically equal groups (A, B and C): random allocation sequence was done through numbered containers. Group A included 22 patients aged between 57 and 74 years (69.2 years old on average), group B included 22 patients aged between 56 and 73 years

(68.8 years old on average), while group C included 22 patients aged between 56 and 74 years (69 years old on average).

Patients were included if they presented presbyacusis with type A tympanogram.

We have considered as exclusion criteria: genetic and congenital condition; neoplasm; acute contemporary bacterial and/or viral ear, upper respiratory tract infections, history of treatment with ototoxic drugs, shooting experiences, systemic disease such as diabetes, any past or present external and/or middle ear infection, history of sudden sensorineural hearing loss and history for occupational or hobby noise exposure.

After signing an informed consent, before and one month after the treatment, all patients undergo the following instrumental examinations: pure tone audiometry, transient evoked otoacoustic emissions (TEAOE) and otoacoustic products of distortion (DPOAE), auditory brainstem response, by MK 12-ABR screener with natus-ALGO2e (Amplifon, Milan, Italy), and vocal audiometry.

At the beginning, a standard 226-Hz probe tone tympanometry was performed in every subject to exclude external and middle ear pathologies.

Tympanograms were defined as type A, B or C according to Jerger [22]: the normal, or type A, tympanogram has a distinct peak in compliance within 0 to - 100 mm of water pressure in the ear canal; with type B tympanogram, there is no peak in compliance but a flat pattern with little or even no apparent change in compliance as a function of pressure in the ear canal; type C tympanogram also has a distinct peak in compliance, but the peak is within the negative pressure region beyond -150 mm of water pressure.

Conventional pure-tone audiometry was carried out in a soundproof room and the pure-tone thresholds of each ear were measured at frequencies of 0.50, 1, 2, 4 and 8 kHz.

TEOAEs and DPOAEs were recorded in a sound-attenuated chamber by an ILO-92 instrument (Amplifon, Milan, Italy): TEOAEs were evoked through a 80- to 85-dB SPL stimuli, with a stimulation rate less than 60 stimuli per second, delivered through a catheter inserted into the external auditory canal. DPOAE were recorded with two acoustic stimuli (pure tones) at 2 frequencies (ie, f1, f2 [f2>f1]) and 2 intensity levels (ie, L1, L2). The acoustic stimuli were simultaneously delivered through a catheter inserted into the external auditory canal, with an automatically determined f2/f1 ratio of 1.22: all DPOAE data were collected for the condition in which $f2$ was fixed at 4 kHz, $f2 / f1 = 1.22$; the level of $f2$ ($L2$) was varied from 20 to 70 dB SPL (in 10-dB steps), and, for each $L2$, $L1$ was set according to the equation, $L1 = 0.4L2 + 39$ dB. The noise level was measured at a frequency of 50 Hz above the DPOAE frequency. For graphic analysis, a plot of mean DPOAE levels was constructed as a function of the stimuli (DP-gram).

Table 1. Pure-tone audiometry results (audiometric air/ audiometric bone thresholds), expressed in dB, at the frequencies of 500 Hz, 1000 Hz, 2000 Hz, 4000 Hz, 8000 Hz before (t=1), at the end (t=2) of the treatment with Q-TER®(P: patient)

P		500 Hz		1000 Hz		2000 Hz		4000 Hz		8000 Hz	
		R	L	R	L	R	L	R	L	R	L
1	t=1	10/5	10/5	10/5	10/5	15/10	10/5	25/25	20/5	15	15
	t=2	0/0	0/0	0/0	0/0	5/0	0/0	25/20	10/5	5	5
2	t=1	15/10	15/10	10/5	5/0	20/15	45/30	40/30	60/55	95	85
	t=2	15/10	15/10	5/0	5/0	20/15	35/30	40/30	60/55	95	85
3	t=1	65/35	65/60	60/35	60/55	85/75	85/80	90/85	90/85	90	90
	t=2	40/35	30/25	45/40	25/20	80/75	75/70	70/85	80/75	90	90
4	t=1	10/5	10/5	10/5	15/10	20/15	15/10	25/20	25/15	30	35
	t=2	10/5	10/5	10/5	15/10	20/15	15/10	20/20	25/20	30	25
5	t=1	0/0	5/0	10/10	15/10	15/15	15/10	15/10	5/0	25	25
	t=2	0/0	5/0	5/0	10/5	5/10	10/10	10/10	5/0	20	20
6	t=1	30/25	45/40	30/25	40/35	40/35	40/35	45/40	60/55	70	75
	t=2	30/25	45/40	30/25	40/30	40/30	35/35	40/35	40/40	70	75
7	t=1	25/20	25/20	40/35	40/35	50/45	50/45	50/45	50/45	85	85
	t=2	20/15	25/20	35/30	40/35	50/45	50/45	50/45	50/45	70	70
8	t=1	15/10	20/15	15/15	20/15	50/45	45/45	70/65	70/65	55	40
	t=2	15/10	15/10	15/10	10/5	45/35	35/30	65/60	65/60	50	40
9	t=1	40/25	45/40	35/30	35/30	25/25	25/25	25/20	25/20	45	45
	t=2	40/10	40/40	25/20	20/10	15/15	20/20	20/10	20/10	45	40
10	t=1	25/20	35/25	25/20	35/30	15/10	25/20	20/10	25/20	20	25
	t=2	25/15	35/15	20/15	30/15	15/10	25/15	20/10	20/15	20	25
11	t=1	35/30	30/25	35/30	30/25	45/40	40/35	45/40	45/40	70	80
	t=2	25/20	20/15	30/25	15/10	40/10	25/20	40/30	35/30	70	40
12	t=1	75/50	60/55	60/50	60/50	60/55	60/55	65/60	60/60	85	85
	t=2	75/50	60/55	60/50	50/45	50/45	50/40	50/45	50/45	70	70
13	t=1	20/20	25/15	20/15	30/20	25/20	30/25	35/30	30/25	60	55
	t=2	20/15	20/15	15/10	20/15	15/10	20/15	35/30	25/20	55	55
14	t=1	25/20	25/20	15/10	15/10	25/20	25/20	35/30	35/30	40	40

Table 1. Continued

	t=2	20/15	20/15	15/10	5/10	15/10	25/20	20/20	20/20	30	30
15	t=1	15/15	15/10	25/20	20/15	35/30	35/30	40/35	35/30	80	80
	t=2	15/15	15/10	25/20	20/15	30/25	20/25	30/25	25/25	80	80
16	t=1	20/15	25/20	20/15	25/20	20/15	20/15	50/45	50/45	75	70
	t=2	10/15	25/20	20/15	20/15	20/15	20/15	45/40	40/40	60	65
17	t=1	20/15	15/10	10/5	15/10	10/5	25/20	35/25	35/30	40	40
	t=2	10/5	15/10	10/5	15/10	10/5	25/20	35/25	35/30	30	30
18	t=1	15/10	15/10	15/10	15/10	25/20	25/20	35/30	40/40	30	30
	t=2	15/10	15/10	15/10	15/10	25/20	25/20	25/20	25/20	30	30
19	t=1	25/15	15/10	25/20	30/15	35/30	35/30	45/40	45/40	50	50
	t=2	20/15	15/10	25/20	20/15	30/25	20/15	30/30	30/30	40	40
20	t=1	20/15	25/20	20/15	25/20	20/15	20/15	50/45	50/45	65	70
	t=2	10/15	25/20	20/15	20/15	20/15	20/15	45/40	50/40	55	70
21	t=1	10/10	15/10	10/5	15/10	25/25	35/30	40/35	40/35	45	45
	t=2	10/5	15/10	10/5	15/10	25/25	35/30	40/35	40/35	35	35
22	t=1	10/5	15/10	10/5	15/10	30/25	35/30	30/5	35/30	35	30
	t=2	10/5	15/10	10/5	15/10	20/20	20/20	30/5	35/30	20	20

Table 2. pure-tone audiometry results (audiometric air/ audiometric bone thresholds), expressed in dB, at the frequencies of 500 Hz, 1000 Hz, 2000 Hz, 4000 Hz, 8000 Hz before (t=1), at the end (t=2) of the treatment with Tocalfa (P: patient)

P		500 Hz		1000 Hz		2000 Hz		4000 Hz		8000 Hz	
		R	L	R	L	R	L	R	L	R	L
1	t=1	5/5	5/5	10/5	10/5	15/10	10/5	25/20	20/5	15	15
	t=2	5/5	5/5	10/5	10/5	15/10	10/5	25/15	20/5	15	15
2	t=1	15/10	15/10	10/5	15/10	20/15	45/30	40/30	60/55	95	85
	t=2	15/10	15/10	10/5	10/10	20/15	40/30	40/30	60/55	90	85
3	t=1	40/35	30/25	30/25	30/25	45/40	45/40	80/75	80/75	80	80
	t=2	40/35	30/25	30/20	25/20	45/40	45/40	70/65	80/75	80	80
4	t=1	10/5	10/5	15/10	15/10	20/15	15/10	25/20	25/15	30	35
	t=2	10/5	10/5	15/10	15/10	20/15	15/10	25/20	25/15	30	25
5	t=1	10/10	15/10	15/10	15/10	15/10	15/10	15/10	15/10	25	25
	t=2	10/10	15/10	15/10	10/5	15/10	10/10	10/10	15/10	25	25

Table 2. Continued

6	t=1	30/25	45/40	35/25	35/35	40/35	45/35	45/40	60/55	60	65
	t=2	30/25	45/40	35/25	35/35	40/35	45/35	45/40	55/50	60	65
7	t=1	25/20	25/20	40/35	40/35	45/45	45/45	50/45	50/45	75	75
	t=2	20/15	25/20	35/30	40/35	45/45	45/45	50/45	50/45	70	75
8	t=1	15/10	20/15	15/15	20/15	45/45	45/35	65/65	65/65	55	50
	t=2	15/10	20/15	15/15	15/15	45/35	45/35	65/60	65/60	55	50
9	t=1	40/35	45/40	45/45	40/40	40/40	40/40	20/10	25/20	45	45
	t=2	40/35	45/40	45/40	40/40	40/40	40/40	20/10	25/20	45	45
10	t=1	25/20	35/25	25/20	35/30	35/30	35/20	20/10	25/20	35	25
	t=2	25/20	35/25	25/20	35/30	35/30	35/20	20/10	25/20	35	25
11	t=1	35/30	30/25	35/30	30/25	45/40	40/35	45/40	45/40	50	50
	t=2	25/30	20/20	30/25	30/25	45/40	40/35	45/40	45/40	50	50
12	t=1	65/60	60/55	80/65	80/65	80/65	80/65	70/55	70/65	85	85
	t=2	65/60	60/55	80/65	80/65	80/65	80/65	70/55	70/65	85	85
13	t=1	20/25	30/20	20/15	30/20	25/20	30/25	35/30	30/25	60	50
	t=2	20/25	30/20	20/15	30/20	25/20	30/25	35/30	30/25	60	50
14	t=1	25/20	25/20	25/20	25/20	25/20	25/20	35/30	35/30	40	40
	t=2	25/20	25/20	25/20	25/20	25/20	25/20	35/30	35/30	40	40
15	t=1	35/35	35/30	35/30	35/30	40/30	40/35	40/35	35/30	40	40
	t=2	35/35	35/30	35/30	35/30	40/30	40/35	40/35	35/30	40	40
16	t=1	20/20	25/20	20/15	25/20	20/15	20/15	40/35	40/35	45	45
	t=2	20/20	25/20	20/15	20/15	20/15	20/15	35/30	35/30	40	45
17	t=1	20/15	20/15	10/5	15/10	25/25	25/20	35/25	35/30	35	35
	t=2	20/15	20/15	10/5	15/10	25/25	25/20	35/25	35/30	35	35
18	t=1	15/10	15/10	15/10	15/10	30/30	30/30	40/35	45/40	35	35
	t=2	15/10	15/10	15/10	15/10	25/20	25/20	40/35	45/40	30	30
19	t=1	25/15	15/10	25/20	30/15	40/35	45/40	50/40	50/40	50	50
	t=2	25/15	15/10	25/20	30/15	40/35	40/40	45/40	45/40	50	50
20	t=1	20/15	25/20	20/15	25/20	40/35	40/35	50/45	50/45	50	50
	t=2	10/15	25/20	20/15	20/20	40/35	40/35	50/45	50/45	50	50
21	t=1	15/10	15/10	20/15	20/15	35/25	35/30	40/35	40/35	40	40
	t=2	10/5	10/10	20/15	20/10	35/25	35/30	40/35	40/35	40	40
22	t=1	20/10	25/20	30/25	30/25	35/30	35/30	40/35	40/35	40	40
	t=2	20/10	25/20	30/25	30/25	35/30	35/30	40/35	40/35	40	40

In vocal audiometry, the vocal material used was composed of lists of phonetically balanced diphonemes.

Group A underwent therapy with Q-TER®, 160 mg, once a day for 30 days; Q-TER® was prepared in sachets.

Group B underwent therapy with vitamin E (50 mg), once a day for 30 days.

Group C received placebo, once a day for 30 days.

In order to maintain double blind conditions, Q-TER®, vitamin E and placebo sachets were identical in shape and size.

Statistical analysis was performed by using a *t* test; probability values less than 0.05 were regarded as significant.

Results

At the end of the treatment in the group A the audiological tests showed:

- an improvement of the mean air and bone audiometric thresholds at the 500 (13/22), 1,000 (15/22), 2,000 (14/22), 4,000 (17/22), and 8,000 Hz (15/22) (Table 1), with regard to the pure-tone audiometry test, in all the patients (22/22);
- the presence of the evoked otoacustic emissions and otoacustic distortion products, which were previously assent at the 800, 1,000, 4,000 and 8,000 Hz (Table 3)

Table 3. DPOAE in patients treated with Q-TER® (P: present; A: assent; t=1: before the treatment; t=2 at the end of the treatment)

P		800 Hz		1000 Hz		4000 Hz		8000 Hz	
		R	L	R	L	R	L	R	L
1	t=1	P	P	P	P	P	P	P	P
	t=2	P	P	P	P	P	P	P	P
2	t=1	P	P	P	P	P	A	A	A
	t=2	P	P	P	P	P	P	A	A
3	t=1	A	A	A	A	A	A	A	A
	t=2	P	P	P	P	A	A	A	A
4	t=1	P	P	P	P	P	P	P	P
	t=2	P	P	P	P	P	P	P	P

Table 3. Continued

5	t=1	P	P	P	P	P	P	P	P
	t=2	P	P	P	P	P	P	P	P
6	t=1	P	P	P	P	P	A	A	A
	t=2	P	P	P	P	P	P	A	A
7	t=1	P	P	P	P	P	P	A	A
	t=2	P	P	P	P	P	P	A	A
8	t=1	P	P	P	P	A	A	A	P
	t=2	P	P	P	P	A	A	A	P
9	t=1	P	P	P	P	P	P	P	P
	t=2	P	P	P	P	P	P	P	P
10	t=1	P	P	P	P	P	P	P	P
	t=2	P	P	P	P	P	P	P	P
11	t=1	P	P	P	P	P	P	A	A
	t=2	P	P	P	P	P	P	A	A
12	t=1	A	A	A	A	A	A	A	A
	t=2	A	A	A	P	P	P	A	A
13	t=1	P	P	P	P	P	P	A	A
	t=2	P	P	P	P	P	P	A	A
14	t=1	P	P	P	P	P	P	P	P
	t=2	P	P	P	P	P	P	P	P
15	t=1	P	P	P	P	P	P	A	A
	t=2	P	P	P	P	P	P	A	A
16	t=1	P	P	P	P	A	A	A	A
	t=2	P	P	P	P	P	P	A	A
17	t=1	P	P	P	P	P	P	P	P
	t=2	P	P	P	P	P	P	P	P
18	t=1	P	P	P	P	P	P	P	P
	t=2	P	P	P	P	P	P	P	P
19	t=1	P	P	P	P	P	P	A	A
	t=2	P	P	P	P	P	P	P	P
20	t=1	P	P	P	P	A	P	A	P
	t=2	P	P	P	P	P	P	P	P
21	t=1	P	P	P	P	P	P	P	P
	t=2	P	P	P	P	P	P	P	P
22	t=1	P	P	P	P	P	P	P	P
	t=2	P	P	P	P	P	P	P	P

At the end of the treatment in the group B the audiological tests showed:

- an improvement of the mean air and bone audiometric thresholds at the 500 (4/22), 1,000 (7/22), 2,000 (4/22), 4,000 (6/22), and 8,000 Hz (3/22) (Table 2), with regard to the pure-tone audiometry test in 12/22 patients;
- the presence of the evoked otoacustic emissions and otoacustic distortion products, which were previously assent at the 800, 1,000, 4,000 and 8,000 Hz. (Table 4)

We found no significant differences in the others parameters and in group C. No patients experienced side effects.

Discussion

Presbycusis is the third most prevalent condition of elderly persons; presbycusis is the result of the combined effects of intrinsic aging of the peripheral and central auditory systems: degeneration of central auditory pathway during aging, with or without associated loss of hair cells, is common in humans and animals [23].

Until now, the pathogenesis of presbycusis is not well understood. One of the current hypotheses is that loss of neurons, at the level of the central auditory pathway, in animals and in humans is secondary to loss of hair cells [24]: numerous studies indicate that the target hair cells release trophic factors that support the central auditory system pathway [25]. After chemical or mechanical damage of hair cells, neurons are rapidly lost, consistent with a target-dependent mechanism of survival [23].

During the aging process, however, the degeneration of central auditory pathway may not arise strictly as a secondary degeneration after hair cell loss, because the extent of the neurons death is much greater than that of hair cells [23]. Likewise, the localization of the neurons loss is not alwa ys correlated with the location of hair cell loss [23]. Thus, the slow loss of neurons during aging may involve hair cell-dependent and -independent mechanisms [26].

Nicotinic acetylcholine receptors (nAChRs) are a multigene family of ligand-gated ion channels that participate in synaptic transmission [27].

Age-related changes of nAChR subunits expression in the central nervous system (CNS) have been well documented [23].

Table 4. DPOAE in patients treated with vitamin E (P: present; A: assent; t=1: before the treatment; t=2 at the end of the treatment)

P		800 Hz		1000 Hz		4000 Hz		8000 Hz	
		R	L	R	L	R	L	R	L
1	t=1	P	P	P	P	P	P	P	P
	t=2	P	P	P	P	P	P	P	P
2	t=1	P	P	P	P	P	A	A	A
	t=2	P	P	P	P	P	A	A	A
3	t=1	P	P	P	P	A	A	A	A
	t=2	P	P	P	P	A	A	A	A
4	t=1	P	P	P	P	P	P	P	P
	t=2	P	P	P	P	P	P	P	P
5	t=1	P	P	P	P	P	P	P	P
	t=2	P	P	P	P	P	P	P	P
6	t=1	P	P	P	P	A	A	A	A
	t=2	P	P	P	P	A	A	A	A
7	t=1	P	P	P	P	A	A	A	A
	t=2	P	P	P	P	A	A	A	A
8	t=1	P	P	P	P	A	A	A	A
9	t=2	P	P	P	P	A	A	A	A
9	t=1	P	P	P	P	P	P	P	P
	t=2	P	P	P	P	P	P	P	P
10	t=1	P	P	P	P	P	P	P	P
	t=2	P	P	P	P	P	P	P	P
11	t=1	P	P	P	P	P	P	A	A
	t=2	P	P	P	P	P	P	A	A
12	t=1	A	A	A	A	A	A	A	A
	t=2	A	A	A	A	A	A	A	A
13	t=1	P	P	P	P	P	P	A	A
	t=2	P	P	P	P	P	P	A	A
14	t=1	P	P	P	P	P	P	P	P
	t=2	P	P	P	P	P	P	P	P
15	t=1	P	P	P	P	P	P	P	P
	t=2	P	P	P	P	P	P	P	P
16	t=1	P	P	P	P	P	P	P	P
	t=2	P	P	P	P	P	P	P	P

Table 4. Continued

17	t=1	P	P	P	P	P	P	P	P
	t=2	P	P	P	P	P	P	P	P
18	t=1	P	P	P	P	P	P	P	P
	t=2	P	P	P	P	P	P	P	P
19	t=1	P	P	P	P	A	A	A	A
	t=2	P	P	P	P	A	A	A	A
20	t=1	P	P	P	P	A	A	A	A
	t=2	P	P	P	P	A	A	A	A
21	t=1	P	P	P	P	P	P	P	P
	t=2	P	P	P	P	P	P	P	P
22	t=1	P	P	P	P	P	P	P	P
	t=2	P	P	P	P	P	P	P	P

The nicotinic acetylcholine receptor (nAChR) is a ligand-gated ion channel that mediates neurotransmission at the neuromuscular junction, autonomic ganglia and at some sites in the central nervous system. Distinct nAChR subtypes exist that can be stimulated by the neurotransmitter acetylcholine, the natural product nicotine, or by synthetic compounds. *nAChR is the prototype for a protein superfamily that includes the receptors for the excitatory amino acids glutamate and aspartate, the inhibitory amino-acids gamma-aminobutyric acid (GABA) and glycine, as well as the serotonin 5-HT₃ receptor* [28].

In recent years, it has become clear that the neuronal nAChR is a valid target against a variety of diseases, including cognitive and attention deficits, Parkinson's disease, anxiety, and pain management [29]; the addiction liability and other undesirable side-effects of nicotine prohibit the use of this natural product for therapeutic applications, but the active development of nAChR agonists presenting adequate receptor subtype specificity should result in improved pharmacology and potency [29].

Several recent studies suggest that, in addition to their traditional role in synaptic transmission, activation of nAChR subunits could protect neurons or lead to neuronal apoptosis [30,31].

The activity of nAChRs is related with NMDA receptors. When complied with NMDA, nAChR is neuroprotective without decreasing the NMDA-mediated (Ca^{2+}) rise [32]. This paradox is generated because depending on the pathway of Ca^{2+} entry, different downstream effectors are activated [33]. Ca^{2+} is one of the main players in the regulation of excitotoxicity and neuronal survival. There are several routes of Ca^{2+} entry into neurons, of which the NMDA receptor, cannot be ignored. nAChR induces Ca^{2+} increase: Ca^{2+} is a second messenger that regulates many processes in the brain. Among others, Ca^{2+} influx modulates cell signaling by activation of mitogen-activated protein kinases, leading to adaptive changes that include activation of transcription factors. One of the branches of mitogen-activated protein kinases, the Raf-MEK-ERK cascade is usually involved in neuroprotection. Neuronal survival is also promoted, in a Ca^{2+}-dependent manner, by phosphatidylinositol 3-kinase (PI 3-kinase) [33,34].

nAChRs can modulate the activity of NMDA receptor and avoid that higher intraplasmatic levels of Ca^{2+} lead to apoptosis. The fact that the neuroprotective effect of nicotine is Ca^{2+}-dependent and effective after NMDA application suggests that nicotine triggers a neuroprotective program involving neurotrophins and protein kinases. Ca^{2+} entry increases the phosphorylation of transcription factors followed by neurotrophin synthesis. There is evidence that neuroprotection mediated by nAChRs involves neurotrophins, as Trk [35].

The survival-promoting activity of the Trk neurotrophin receptors involves, among others, the docking of adapter proteins that activate Ras. Ras activates the PI-3 kinase and the Raf-1, MEK, ERK kinase cascade [36].

It has been reported that the cell death and/or neurotoxicity is related to the cellular accumulation of calcium: the elevation in calcium accounts for a mitochondrial dysfunction [37].

Moreover, evidence indicates that mitochondrial impairment can lead to the release of cytochrome c from mitochondria into the cytoplasm. This release may occur with the treatment of cells with many apoptotic stimuli. On entry into the cytosol, cytochrome c binds the caspase-activating protein Apaf-1, stimulating its binding to pro-caspase 9 and activating caspase networks that activate apoptosis [38].

Another important finding is that the neuroprotection conferred by nAChRs activation may be mediated through the mitochondrial retention of cytochrome c. This finding is consistent with a recent publications which reported that nicotine, acting through the alpha7 receptor, can protect against mitochondrial dysfunction, cytochrome c release and caspase activation in cultured spinal cord neurons [30].

Therefore, one of the potential mechanisms by which activation of the alpha7 nicotinic receptor can protect against induced alterations in mitochondrial potential and cytochrome c release, could be the activation of protein kinase C and increased activation of bcl-2 [39].

CoQ10 is a vitamin-like antioxidant that reacts with oxygen radicals and lipoperoxides to prevent damage to biomolecules in various tissues and cell compartments. It is found in highest concentrations in tissues with high-energy turnover such as the heart, brain, liver and kidney. And as other antioxidants like vitamin E, vitamine C, and idebenone, CoQ10 is studied for several kinds of sensorineural hearing loss including noise-induced hearing loss [40].

The mechanisms of CoQ10 in inner ear are reported in several experimental studies. The mechanisms of cochlear damage due to various causes are related to lipid oxidation, protein oxidation, and DNA damage. CoQ10 inhibits inner ear lipid peroxidation by either scavenging free radicals directly or by reducing α-tocopheroxyl radical to α-tocopherol. CoQ10 also protects proteins and DNA from oxidation [40,41].

And recently, water-soluble CoQ10 was developed to improve absorption of CoQ10,and in several studies using water-soluble CoQ10 in guinea pigs, showed to reduce cochlear oxidative stress induced by noise [17].

Clinically, Angeli et al. reported that CoQ10 may be helpful in delaying the progression of hearing loss in patients with the 7445A→G mitochondrial mutation [16].

Suzuki et al. also reported similar results in patients with maternally inherited diabetes mellitus and deafness due to the mtDNA 3243A→G mutation [42]. And, according to Cadoni et al., serum levels of CoQ10 was significantly lower in SSNHL patients than control group [43].

In our experience, treatment with Q-TER® and/or Vit E was very effective in the prevention of neural damage in presbycusis. It is known that Q-TER® induces an elevation of Vit E concentration in tissues of rats and it is known, that the rate of O^2 elimination is directly related to the Vit E concentration, indicating the role of Vit E in the elimination of radicals

At the same time, Q-TER® has an important role in the prevention of lipid peroxidation and oxidative damage of tissues, and thus induces changes in the activity of many enzymes [13, 41].

Our results are consistent with recent studies where it has been hypothesized that a water formulation of CoQ10 inhibits apoptosis in human neuronal cells challenged with glutamate excitotoxicity or hydrogen peroxide or paraquat induced oxidative stress [44].

It is well known that mitochondria are in the centre of the intrinsic pathway of apoptosis, and it has been recently demonstrated that soluble multicomposite of CoQ10 decreased the number of apoptotic cells, prevented mitochondrial depolarization and stabilized mitochondrial membrane and inhibited cytocrome c release [17]. Because the therapeutic approach with CoQ10 is limited by its poor bioavailability in aqueous media, Q-TER®, compared with CoQ10, presents an higher level of protection [17].

The side effects for administration of CoQ10 is very rare, mainly mild gastrointestinal discomfort is reported in less than 1% of patients in clinical trials.

But in this study, gastrointestinal discomfort may have been masked, because antacid andantiulcerant was routinely prescribed to reduce gastrointestinal discomfort induced by oral steroids. Other rare toxicities such as rash, irritability, headache, heartburn, and fatigue was also reported, but was not seen in this study. No absolute contraindication is reported for CoQ10, but potential interactions with warfarin and statins have been suggested in case studies [45,46].

In clinical studies of various fields, dose usage of CoQ10 ranges from 30mg to 3000mg per day. Prescription pattern also differs from once a day to three times a day, and as short as 2 weeks to as long as a year in Parkison's disease. Acceptable daily intake for CoQ10 is reported as 12 mg/kg/day (so, 720mg/day in an adult person weighing 60 kg).

Because compared to native CoQ10, Q-TER® is about 200 times more soluble in water, allowing a greater bioavailability and an improved chemical stability compared to native form, we have used a dosage of 160mg/day for 30 days.

Although these preliminary data are positive, because the small number of patients treated, further studies are needed to determine therapeutic doses and durations that induces better hearing improvement in presbyacusis [46].

Conclusion

The preliminary data presented in this study are encouraging for a larger clinical trial to collect additional evidence on the effect of Q-TER® in preventing the development of hearing loss in subjects with presbyacusis.

Our experience highlights the effectiveness of this product in inducing neuroplasticity in elderly.

References

[1]   Kalivas P.W. & O'Brien C. (2008). Drug addition as a pathology of staged neuroplasticity. *Neuropsychopharmacology*, 33, 166-80.

[2]   Hyman, SE; Malenka, RC; Nestler, EJ. Neural mechanisms of addiction: the role of reward-related learning and memory. Annu Rev Neurosci, 2006, 29: 565–598.

[3]   Kalivas P.W. & Volkow N.D. (2005). The neural basis of addiction: a pathology of motivation and choice. *Am J Psychiatry*, 162, 1403–1413.

[4]   Wrang, L-Y. The dynamic range for gain control of NMDA receptor-mediated synaptic transmission at a single synapse. *The journal of neuroscience*, 2000, 20.

[5]   Zheng W. & Knudsen E.I. (1999). Functional selection of adaptive auditory space map by GABAA – mediated inhibition. *Science*, 284, 962-65.

[6]   Nestler EJ. Is there a common molecular pathway for addiction? *Nat Neurosci*, 2005, 8, 1445–1449.

[7]   Kalivas P.W. The glutamate homeostasis hypothesis of addiction. *Nature Reviewers Neuroscience*, 2009, 10: 561-572.

[8]   Kalivas P.W. How do we determine which drug-induced neuroplastic changes are important? *Nature Reviewers Neuroscience*, 2005, 11, 1440-41.

[9]   Wang, KK; Larner, SF; Robinson, G; Hayes, RL. Neuroprotection targets after traumatic brain injury. *Curr Opin Neurol*, 2006, 19: 514–519.

[10]   Muresanu, FD; Buia, MR; Pintea, D; Craiovan,S; Moldovan, F; Opincariu, I; Maslarov, D; Stan, A. Neuroprotection and neuroplasticity in craniocerebral trauma. *Romanian Journal of Neurology*, 2007, 4, 2007, 154-165.

[11]   Moschetti, T; Giuffrè, A; Ardiccioni, C; Vallone, B; Modjtahedi, N; Kroemer, G; Brunori, M. Failure of apoptosis-inducing factor to act as neuroglobin reductase. *Biochem Biophys Res Commun*, 2009, 390: 121-4.

[12]   Droge W. Free radicals in the physiological control of cell function. *Physiol Rev*, 2002, 82, 47-95.

[13]   Chen H. & Tappel A.L. (1995). Protection by vitamin E, selenium, trolox C, ascorbic acid palmitate, acetylcysteine, coenzyme Q0, coenzyme Q10, beta-carotene, canthaxantine, and (+)-catechin against oxidative damage to rat blood and tissues in vivo. *Free Radical Biol Med*, 1995, 18, 949-53.

[14]   Crane F.L. Biochemical functions of coenzyme Q10. *J Am Coll Nutr*, 2001, 20, 591-98.

[15]   Lass A. & Sohal R.S. (2000). Effect of coenzyme Q10 and -tocopherol content of mitochondria on the production of superoxide anion radicals. *FASEB J*, 14, 87- 94.

[16]   Angeli, SI; Liu, XZ; Yan, D; Balkany, T; Telischi, F. Coenzyme Q-10 treatment of patients with a 7445A--->G mitochondrial DNA mutation stops the progression of hearing loss. *Acta Otolaryngol* 2005, 125, 510-512.

[17]   Fetoni, AR; Piacentini, R; Fiorita, A; Paludetti, G; Troiani, D. Water-soluble Coenzyme Q10 formulation (Q-ter) promotes outer hair cell survival in a guinea pig model of noise induced hearing loss (NIHL). *Brain Res*, 2009, 1257, 108-116.

[18] Sato K. Pharmacokinetics of coenzyme Q10 in recovery of acute sensorineural hearing loss due to hypoxia. *Acta Otolaryngol Supp* 1988, 458, 95-102.

[19] Ibrahim, WH; Blagavan, HN; Chopra, RK; Chow CK. Dietary coenzyme Q10 and vitamin E alter the status of these compounds in rat tissues and mitochondria. *J Nutr*, 2000, 130, 2343-49.

[20] Fetoni, AR; Garzaro, M; Ralli, M; Landolfo, V; Sensini, M; Pecorari, G; Mordente, A; Paludetti, G; Giordano, C. The monitoring role of otoacoustic emissions and oxidative stress markers in the protective effects of antioxidant administration in noise-exposed subjects: a pilot study. Med Sci Monit 2009, 15, PR 1-8.

[21] Corvi Mora, P; Canal, T; Fortuna, F; Ruzzier, F. Composition containing micronutrients with improved anti-oxidant activity and use thereof. WO/2007/009997.

[22] Jerger, JF. Clinical experience with impedence audiometry. *Arch Otolaryngol*, 1970, 92, 11-24.

[23] Bao,J; Lei, D; Du,Y; Ohlemiller,K.K; Beaudet, A.L.; Role, LW. Requirement of Nicotinic Acetylcholine Receptor Subunit β2 in the Maintenance of Spiral Ganglion Neurons during Aging. *The Journal of Neuroscience*, 2005, 25, 3041–3045.

[24] Keithley E.M. & Croskrey K.L. (1990). Spiral ganglion cell endings in the cochlear nucleus of young and old rats. *Hear Res,* 49, 169 –177.

[25] Hossain, WA; Brumwell, CL; Morest, DK. Sequential interactions of fibroblast growth factor-2, brain-derived neurotrophic factor, neurotrophin-3, and their receptors define critical periods in the development of cochlear ganglion cells. *Exp Neurol*, 2002, 175, 138 –151.

[26] Ohlemiller K.K. & Gagnon P.M. (2004). Apical-to-basal gradients in age-related cochlear degeneration and their relationship to "primary" loss of coclea neurons. *J Comp Neurol,* 479, 103-116.

[27] McGehee, D.S. & Role, L.W. (1995). Physiological diversity of nicotinic acetylcholine receptors expressed by vertebrate neurons. *Annu Rev Physiol*, 57, 521–546.

[28] Changeux, JP; Bertrand, D; Corringer, PJ; Dehaene, S; Edelstein, S; Lena, C; Le Novere, N; Marubio, L; Picciotto, M; Zoli, M. Brain nicotinic receptors: structure and regulation, role in learning and reinforcement. *Brain Res Rev,* 1998, 26, 198-216.

[29] Lloyd G.K. & Williams M. (2000). Neuronal nicotinic acetylcholine receptors as novel drug targets. *J. Pharmacol Exp Ther*, 292, 461-7.

[30] Garrido, R; Mattson, M.P.; Hennig, B; Toborek, M. Nicotine protects against arachidonic-acid-induced caspase activation, cytochrome c release and apoptosis of cultured spinal cord neurons. J Neurochem, 2001, 76:1395–1403.

[31] Gotti C. & Clementi F. (2004). Neuronal nicotinic receptors: from structure to pathology. *Prog Neurobiol*, 74, 363–396.

[32] Dajas-Bailador, FA; Lima, PA; Wonnacott, S. The α7 nicotinic acetylcholine receptor subtype mediates nicotine protection against NMDA excitotoxicity in primary hippocampal cultures through a Ca^{2+} dependent mechanism. *Neuropharmacology,* 2000, 39, 2799–2807.

[33] Ferchmin, PA; Perez, D; Eterovic, VA; De Vellis, J. Nicotinic receptors differentially regulate N-Methyl-Daspartate damage in acute hippocampal slices. *The J of pharmacology and experimental therapeutics,* 2003, 305, 1971-78.

[34] Perkinton, MS; Ip, JK; Wood, GL; Crossthwaite, AJ; Williams, RJ. Phosphatidylinositol 3-kinase is a central mediator of NMDA receptor signaling to MAP kinase (Erk1/2), Akt/PKB and CREB in striatal neurons. *J Neurochem*, 2002, 80, 239–254.

[35] Belluardo, N; Mudo, G; Blum, M; Fuxe, K. Central nicotinic receptors, neurotrophic factors and neuroprotection. *Behav Brain Res, 2000,* 113, 21–34.

[36] Patapoutian A. & Reichardt L.F. (2001). Trk receptors: mediators of neurotrophin action. *Curr Opin Neurobiol,* 11, 272–280.

[37] Li, Y; King, MA; Meyer, EM. Alpha7 nicotinic receptor mediated protection against ethanol-induced oxidative stress and cytotoxicity in PC12 cells. Brain Res, 2000, 861, 165–167.

[38] Krajewski, S; Krajewska, M; Ellerby, LM; Reed JC. Release of caspase-9 from mitochondria during neuronal apoptosis and cerebral ischemia. *Proc. Natl Acad Sci USA*, 1999, 96, 5752–5757.

[39] Li, Y; Meyer, EM; Alker, WW; Millard, WJ; He, YJ; King, MA. Alpha7 nicotinic receptor activation inhibits ethanol-induced mitochondrial dysfunction, cytochrome c release and neurotoxicity in primary rat hippocampal neuronal cultures. *Journal of Neurochemistry*, 2002, 81, 853–858.

[40] Hirose, Y; Sugahara, K; Mikuriya, T; Hashimoto, M; Shimogori, H; Yamashita, H. Effect of water-soluble coenzyme Q10 on noise-induced hearing loss in guinea pigs. *Acta Otolaryngol* 2008, 128, 1071-1076.

[41] Morimitsu, T; Hagiwara, T; Ide, M; Matsumoto, I; Okada, S. Effect of intermittent sound stimulation on cochlear microphonics and the possible preventive effect of coenzyme Q10. *Hear Res,* 1980, 155-166.

[42] Suzuki, S; Hinokio, Y; Ohtomo, M; Hirai, M; Hirai, A; Chiba, M; Kasuga, S; Satoh, Y; Akai, H; Toyota, T. The effects of coenzyme Q10 treatment on maternally inherited diabetes mellitus and deafness, and mitochondrial DNA 3243 (A to G) mutation. *Diabetologia,* 1998, 41, 584-588.

[43] Cadoni, G; Scipione, S; Agostino, S; Addolorato, G; Cianfrone, F; Leggio, L; Paludetti, G; Lippa, S. Coenzyme Q 10 and cardiovascular risk factors in idiopathic sudden sensorineural hearing loss patients. *Otol Neurotol* 2007;28:878-83.

[44] Sandhu, JK; Pandey, S; Ribecco-Lutkiewicz, M; Monette, R; Borowy-Borowski, H; Walker, PR; Sirkoska, M. Molecular mechanisms of glutamate neurotoxicity in mixed cultures of NT2-derived neurons and astrocytes: protective effects of coenzyme Q10. *J Neurosci Res,* 2003, 72, 691-703.

[45] Ernster L- & Dallner G. (1995). Biochemical, physiological and medical aspects of ubiquinone function. *Biochem Biophys Acta,* 1271, 195-204.

[46] Hidaka, T; Fujii, K; Funahashi, I; Fukutomi, N; Hosoe, K. Safety assessment of coenzyme Q10 (CoQ10). *Biofactors,* 2008, 32, 199-208.

In: Neuroplasticity in the Auditory Brainstem   ISBN 978-1-61761-949-6
Editor: Angelo Salami, pp. 143-170   © 2011 Nova Science Publishers, Inc.

Chapter IX

Central Auditory System Neuroplasticity and Hippocampal Neurogenesis following Cochlear Insults

B. L. Allman, W. Sun, K. S. Kraus, D. Ding,
G. D. Chen, D. Stolzberg, E. Lobarinas, and R. Salvi*

Center for Hearing and Deafness, 137 Cary Hall, State University of New
York at Buffalo, 3435 Main Street, Buffalo, NY 14214, USA

Abstract

Sensorineural hearing loss from noise exposure and ototoxic drugs has
traditionally been thought of as an exclusively cochlear phenomenon because
of compelling evidence of damage to the hair cells and spiral ganglion
neurons. However, there is growing evidence that cochlear pathology leads
to a plethora of functional and subtle anatomical changes at multiple sites
along the auditory pathway as well significant changes in other sensory

* Corresponding author: Richard Salvi, Center for Hearing and Deafness, 137 Cary Hall,
University at Buffalo, Buffalo, NY 14214, Phone: 716 829 5310, Fax: 716 829 2980,
Email: salvi@buffalo.edu

systems and non-auditory regions of the central nervous system. Here we review some of the striking electrophysiological, behavioral and neuroanatomical changes that occur following various cochlear insults. A common theme that emerges from these studies is that cochlear damage, which reduces the neural output of the cochlea, often leads to sound-evoked hyperactivity along the auditory pathway, particularly at the auditory cortex, as well as behavioral evidence of hyperactivity. Surprisingly, noise-induced cochlear damage has a significant impact on cell proliferation and neurogenesis in the hippocampus, a region of the brain involved in memory and spatial navigation. The logical conclusion from decades of research is that peripheral hearing loss has profound effects on the function of the central auditory system.

Introduction

The mammalian inner ear contains two anatomically and functionally distinct types of hair cells: inner hair cells (IHCs), whose innervation by type I spiral ganglion neurons provide the transmission of acoustic information to the central auditory system via the auditory nerve, and outer hair cells (OHCs), which increase the sound sensitivity and frequency selectivity of the inner ear. Given the functional specificity of the IHCs and OHCs, it is not surprising that damage confined to only one hair cell population has a distinct effect on the quality of information entering the central auditory system. For example, selective damage to the IHCs reduces the number of auditory nerve fibers capable of responding to acoustic stimuli (i.e., the central auditory system does not receive the full complement of information), yet the auditory nerve fibers contacting the surviving IHCs still display normal thresholds and sharp tuning properties (i.e., the quality of their information is not altered) [Wang et al., 1997]. In contrast, when cochlear damage is limited to the OHCs, there is an elevation of threshold and a loss of frequency selectivity in the information transmitted by type I auditory nerve fibers [Ryan and Dallos 1975; Dallos and Harris 1978; Ryan et al., 1979; Schmiedt et al., 1980]. In this case, the central auditory system receives input from the full complement of auditory nerve fibers, but their sensitivity and tuning is significantly impaired. Both scenarios result in a decrease in the neural input to the central auditory system irrespective of functional differences following selective hair cell loss.

For the past several years, our research has focused on the morphological and functional changes that occur in the peripheral and central auditory system after various cochlear insults. Using animal models, we have investigated neuroplasticity in the central auditory system induced by a variety of ototraumatic agents: (1) high doses of salicylate, the anti-inflammatory component of aspirin known to cause transient hearing loss, (2) carboplatin, a commonly-used ototoxic chemotherapy drug, and (3) acoustic overstimulation (i.e., noise exposure). In addition to assessing the extent of cochlear damage with histological techniques and hair cell counts (cochleograms), we have used a system-level approach to study the neuroanatomical, electrophysiological and behavioral consequences of neuroplasticity in the auditory pathway caused by the aforementioned cochlear insults. From our collective studies, a consistent theme has emerged: despite decreased neural output from the damaged cochlea, neuroplasticity in the central auditory system often results in sound-evoked cortical hyperactivity. We speculate that cortical hyperactivity following hearing loss may contribute to the aberrant auditory perception that often accompanies cochlear insults, such as tinnitus (i.e., phantom sound perception) and hyperacusis (i.e., marked intolerance to ordinary environmental sound). The following sections will summarize our work on central auditory system neuroplasticity induced by salicylate intoxication, carboplatin ototoxicity, and acoustic overstimulation. Finally, we will present our recent findings on the negative effect of acoustic overstimulation on neurogenesis in the hippocampus; evidence that suggests that noise exposure not only affects the auditory pathway but also non-classical auditory regions of the central nervous system important for higher cognitive processing.

Salicylate-Induced Cochlear Insult

It is well documented that a high-dose of salicylate reliably induces transient hearing loss in humans and laboratory animals (for review, see [Cazals 2000]). This elevation of hearing threshold has been ascribed to a reduction in OHC electromotility and the resulting decrease in neural output from the cochlea [Brownell 1990; Tunstall et al., 1995; Muller et al., 2003; Ermilov et al., 2005; Zhi et al., 2007; Ruel et al., 2008]. For both humans and laboratory animals, electromotility of the OHCs can be assessed non-invasively using the distortion product otoacoustic emission (DPOAE). Following a single high-dose of salicylate, there is a reduction in the amplitude of the DPOAE, indicative of cochlear dysfunction [Huang et al., 2005; Ralli et al., 2010]. Paradoxically, following sessation of chronic exposure to high-doses of salicylate, there is an enhancement of the DPOAE [Huang et al., 2005; Chen et al., 2010], associated with increased OHC electromotility and elevated expression of prestin, the electromechanical protein of OHCs [Yang et al., 2009]. While high-doses of salicylate have traditionally been thought to only affect the cochlea, our recent studies indicate that salicylate induces unexpected functional changes in the central auditory system [Yang et al., 2007; Sun et al., 2009]. Furthermore, we have found that prolonged exposure to high-doses of salicylate cause permanent functional deficits in the auditory pathway [Chen et al., 2010].

Acute Salicylate Exposure

The effects of acute salicylate intoxication on the auditory system have been studied for many years. Recently, we demonstrated an enhancement of the sound-evoked responses in the auditory cortex (AC) of rats 2-hours after a single systemic injection of salicylate [Yang et al., 2007]. To determine if this salicylate-induced AC hyperactivity originated in the cochlea, inferior colliculus (IC) or AC, we performed a follow-up study in which salicylate was administered systemically (250 mg/kg, i.p.) or applied directly to the round window in the middle ear (~50 µl, 25 mg/ml) [Sun et al., 2009]. Electrodes implanted in the IC and AC recorded the amplitude of sound-evoked local field potentials (ICP and ACP, respectively), and an electrode placed on the round window recorded the cochlear compound action potential (CAP). Salicylate administered either systemically or directly to the round window resulted in a decrease in the amplitude of the CAP (Figure 1A, 1B), indicative of a reduction of the summed neural input to the central auditory pathway. Despite these similar results at the level of the auditory nerve, the two salicylate treatments differed profoundly in their effect on the neural responses recorded in the IC and AC. Similar to our previous study [Yang et al., 2007], 1-hour after a systemic injection of salicylate there was a marked increase in the ACP amplitude, suggestive of increased gain in the central auditory system (Figure 1E). Given that the ICP amplitude was essentially unchanged after salicylate treatment (Figure 1C) while the output of the cochlea (CAP) was reduced (Figure 1A), these results imply that a portion of the system gain observed at the level of the AC is likely already manifested between the cochlea and the IC. In contrast, following salicylate application to the round window, there was a reduction in the sound-evoked potentials recorded from both the IC and AC (Figure 1D, 1F). Because the round window application of salicylate caused a decrease in the ACP amplitude, reflecting the reduced peripheral input, the enhancement of the AC response observed after the systemic injection could not be due solely to cochlear mechanisms.

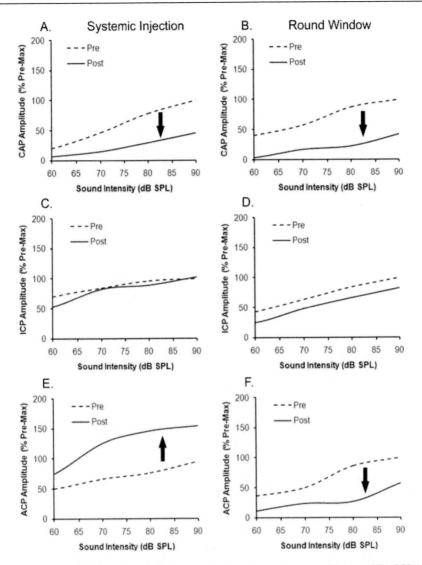

Figure 1. Schematic illustrating typical amplitude-level functions for CAP (A and B), ICP (C and D) and ACP (E and F) recorded before (pre) and one-hour after (post) salicylate was administered systemically (left column) or applied directly to the round window (right column) in the rat. Amplitudes are normalized to the maximum pre-treatment response. Both treatments resulted in a decrease in the CAP amplitude (A and B); however, unlike the direct application (F), there was a significant increase in the ACP amplitude following the systemic injection (E), indicative of an increase in central gain. Arrows show the direction of amplitude change at moderate- to high-intensities. [Sun et al., 2009].

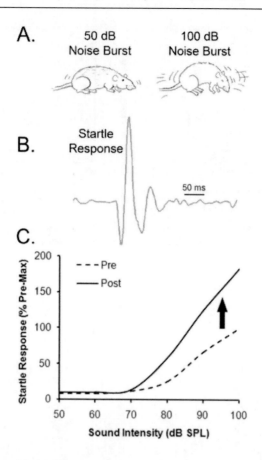

Figure 2. Acoustic startle responses were recorded before (pre) and one-hour after (post) salicylate was administered systemically in the rat. (A) The acoustic startle reflex behavioral paradigm assesses the abrupt motor movement following a loud sound. (B) An example of a startle response recorded from a rat. (C) Schematic illustrating typical startle response amplitudes at various sound intensities pre- and post-salicylate. Startle responses are normalized to the maximum pre-treatment response. One-hour after salicylate, the startle response amplitude at high-intensities increased significantly (arrow), indicative of hyperacusis-behavior. [Sun et al., 2009].

Collectively, our findings suggest that, in addition to causing a reduction in neural output from the cochlea, salicylate exerts a direct effect on the response properties of neurons in the auditory pathway. In support of this hypothesis, Wang and colleagues [Wang et al., 2006] found, using whole-cell patch clamp recording techniques in vitro, that salicylate reduced the inhibitory postsynaptic currents in AC brain slices. Therefore, it is possible that a loss of cortically-mediated inhibition contributed to the AC hyperactivity we observed in vivo. A follow-up in vitro study by Wang and colleagues [Wang et al., 2008] revealed that salicylate also disrupted GABAergic (inhibitory) synaptic transmission in the IC. Finally, in vivo, we demonstrated that salicylate administered systemically failed to induce AC hyperactivity when rats were under isoflurane anesthesia [Sun et al., 2009], which is known to enhance GABA-mediated neurotransmission while suppressing glutamatergic (excitatory) synaptic activity [Neumahr et al., 2000; Ranft et al., 2004]. Apparently, the isoflurane-induced enhancement of GABAergic activity presumably offset the effects of salicylate on the AC. Based on the results of these studies, it appears that salicylate alters the balance of excitation and inhibition in the central auditory system, ultimately leading to AC hyperactivity.

It has been proposed that an increase in central gain resulting from cochlear damage may underlie tinnitus and hyperacusis [Gerken 1996; Salvi et al., 2000; Eggermont and Roberts 2004]. Because salicylate intoxication provides a highly reliable method to insult the cochlea and induce tinnitus, many animal studies have used this model to investigate the neural basis of phantom auditory perception. Our recent study [Sun et al., 2009], however, was the first to investigate whether intolerance to loud sounds (i.e., hyperacusis) is the behavioral correlate of the salicylate-induced AC enhancement. To investigate this possibility, we measured the amplitude of the acoustic startle reflex before and after systemic salicylate administration. The acoustic startle reflex behavioral paradigm exploits an animal's abrupt motoric response to a sudden, loud, startle-eliciting sound (Figure 2A). As described in our recent study [Sun et al., 2009], the rat was placed in a custom-fabricated wire mesh cage that rested on a Plexiglas floor. The startle-eliciting sound (50 ms broadband noise burst presented at six intensities from 50 to 100 dB SPL) was delivered by a loudspeaker located above the cage. A piezoelectric transducer attached to the bottom of the test platform generated a voltage proportional to the magnitude of the startle response (Figure 2B). We found that one hour following systemic salicylate administration the amplitude of the startle response was elevated at sound intensities above 70 dB SPL (Figure 2C). Turner and Parrish [Turner and Parrish 2008] reported a similar salicylate-induced exaggeration of the startle response. It has been suggested that an increase in the startle amplitude is indicative of hyperacusis [Ison et al., 2007]. Because we observed an enhanced startle response over the same range of sound intensities and time as AC hyperactivity [Sun et al., 2009], we propose that intolerance to loud sounds represents a behavioral correlate of the transient neuroplasticity induced by acute salicylate exposure.

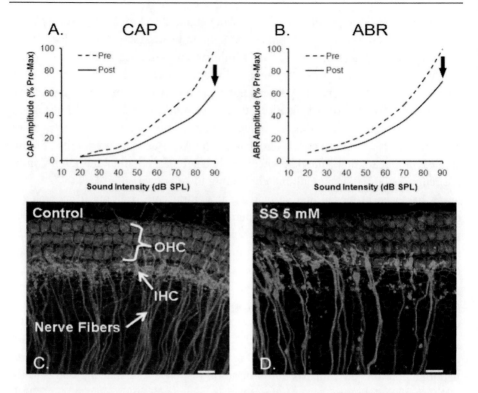

Figure 3. Functional and structural effects of salicylate exposure. (A and B) Schematics illustrating typical amplitude-level functions for CAP (A) and ABR (B) recorded before (pre) and 4-weeks after (post) chronic high-dose salicylate exposure in rat. Amplitudes are normalized to the maximum pre-treatment response. The CAP and ABR amplitudes were reduced post-treatment, suggestive of a functional deficit in the auditory pathway induced by prolonged exposure to high-doses of salicylate. Arrows indicate the direction of amplitude change at high-intensities. [Chen et al., 2010]. (C and D) Typical confocal micrographs of control and salicylate-treated (SS) cochlear organotypic cultures from immature rat showing the hair cells and spiral ganglion nerve fibers. Although the hair cells (OHCs or IHCs) were undamaged, 48 hours of exposure to 5 mM of salicylate significantly reduced the number of nerve fiber fascicles. [Wei et al., 2010].

Chronic Salicylate Exposure

Although aspirin is one of the most widely used drugs, our recent study [Chen et al., 2010] represents one of the few investigations into the effect of chronic high-dose salicylate exposure on the sensorineural properties in the auditory system. Similar to a previous report [Huang et al., 2005], we observed an increase in DPOAE amplitude after chronic salicylate exposure. During this time of enhanced OHC motility, however, we found a reduction in the amplitude of the CAP and auditory brainstem response (ABR), a measure of the sound-evoked neural activity in the brainstem as recorded from subdermal electrodes (Figure 3A, 3B). It appears these deficits were permanent, as they persisted for the duration of our post-treatment testing (four weeks). Because we found no evidence of OHC loss nor a long-term reduction in the DPOAE, we hypothesized the reduction in the CAP amplitude resulted from chronic salicylate-induced damage to the neurites, soma or axons of the spiral ganglion neurons (SGNs). In support of this hypothesis, our follow-up study [Wei et al., 2010] on immature rat cochlear organotypic cultures revealed a salicylate-induced loss of peripheral nerve fibers and severe shrinkage of SGN soma (Figure 3D), indicative of cells undergoing apoptosis [Wyllie et al., 1980; Bortner and Cidlowski 1998; Maeno et al., 2000; Okada et al., 2001; Friis et al., 2005]. These findings were in agreement with a previous in vitro study in which salicylate damaged the spiral ganglion neurites, but not hair cells [Gao 1999]. Based on our in vivo and in vitro results, we suggest that long-term administration of high-doses of salicylate may exert neurotoxic effects on adult SGNs that cause a reduction of neural input to the central auditory system.

Given the modest decrease in the ABR amplitude we observed following chronic salicylate administration (Figure 3B) [Chen et al., 2010], it is reasonable to suspect that, unlike acute exposure (as described above), there may be a reduction in the sound-evoked responses in the AC (i.e., no increase in central gain) after long-term dosing. At present, however, it remains uncertain whether chronic salicylate exposure results in AC hyperactivity and an increased startle response indicative of hyperacusis. It is worth noting that any SGN loss or auditory nerve fiber dysfunction associated with long-term treatment of salicylate would likely exert little effect on behavioral hearing thresholds, but could contribute to poor speech perception or impaired temporal resolution [Schuknecht 1994; Starr et al., 1996].

Carboplatin-induced Ototoxicity

Carboplatin (cis-diamine-l,l-cyclobutane dicarboxylate platinum(II), CBDCA) is a platinum-based, anti-cancer agent known to be cytotoxic to hair cells. In the guinea pig, carboplatin preferentially destroys OHCs [Saito et al., 1989]. In contrast, in the chinchilla, IHCs are more vulnerable to carboplatin exposure than OHCs (Figure 4) [Wake et al., 1994; Trautwein et al., 1996;

Hofstetter et al., 1997; Ding et al., 1999]. To demonstrate the time-course of this unique pattern of hair cell loss, we applied carboplatin directly to the round window of chinchillas (5 mg/ml; 50 μl) and assessed the structural changes at regular time intervals out to 28-days post-treatment [Zhou et al., 2009]. As shown in the schematic cochleogram in Figure 4C, at 3-days post-treatment IHC loss was substantially greater than OHC loss, with the greatest loss of both hair cell types in the basal half of the cochlea. Cochleograms were similar between the 7-day and 14-day time points, where there was 90-100% loss of IHC over the majority of the cochlea (Figure 4D, 4E). Finally, at 28-days post-treatment, there was an increase in OHC loss, such that the surviving hair cells were largely confined to the apical third of the cochlea (Figure 4F). Collectively, these results indicate that the time-course of hair cell loss occurred in two phases: an early phase of rapid hair cell loss, followed by a slow, progressive phase over the next 2-4 weeks.

To determine whether intrinsic and/or extrinsic apoptotic cell death pathways initiated this hair cell loss, we assessed the pattern of caspase activation following direct application of carboplatin on the round window [Zhou et al., 2009]. More specifically, 24-hours after carboplatin treatment, fluorescently-labeled caspase probes, which were capable of detecting activated caspases in living hair cells, were injected into the perilymph. One hour after injection, the cochlea was harvested and the organ of Corti evaluated under a confocal laser scanning microscope. Using appropriate filters, we observed many hair cell nuclei in the basal turn of the cochlea that were abnormally condensed and/or fragmented, indicative of cells in the early stages of apoptosis, and these cells were labeled with cellular membrane caspase-8 and executioner caspase-3, but not mitochondrial caspase-9. Thus, our results confirmed that the loss of hair cells induced by carboplatin exposure was initiated by the extrinsic cell death pathway involving caspase-8 followed by caspase-3, and not an intrinsic cell death pathway initiated by caspase-9.

Unlike the massive loss of both IHCs and OHCs following direct application of carboplatin on the cochlea (described above), a moderate dose of carboplatin delivered systemically to chinchillas results in selective IHC loss along the entire length of the cochlea, with no damage to the OHCs [Hofstetter et al., 1997; Ding et al., 1999]. Given that this pattern of hair cell loss causes a decrease in the output from the cochlea, we asked: how does the central auditory system respond to such partial sensory deprivation? To answer this question, sound-evoked potentials were measured from electrodes implanted at the round window (CAP), IC (ICP) and AC (ACP) before and up to 5 weeks after systemic injection of carboplatin [Qiu et al., 2000]. Figure 5 shows schematics of the typical effects seen in the periphery and central auditory system. Not surprisingly, when ~50% of the IHCs were lost, the CAP amplitude was reduced ~50% at all intensities

(Figure 5A). Despite this dramatic reduction of input to the central auditory system, there was almost no amplitude reduction in the ICP at low to moderate intensities, and much less than a 50% decrease in amplitude at high intensities (Figure 5B). These disparate effects (CAP vs. ICP) suggest that some degree of neuroplasticity had occurred in the brainstem, ultimately increasing the gain of the system to offset the peripheral insult. Furthermore, we observed that the carboplatin-induced neuroplasticity also occurred above the IC, as the ACP amplitude was enhanced in the weeks after the carboplatin treatment (Figure 5C). Thus, additional neural plasticity and enhanced gain may be occurring between the IC and AC.

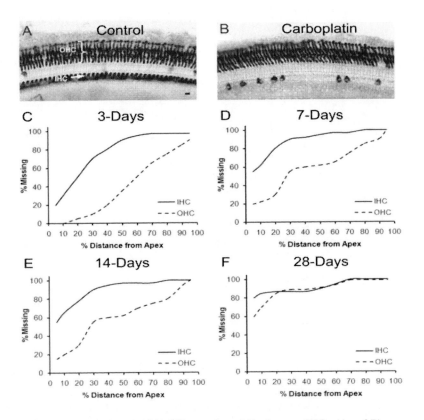

Figure 4. Carboplatin exposure in chinchillas preferentially destroys IHCs. (A and B) Photomicrographs of cochlea before (control) and 1-day after carboplatin application on the round window. Notice the selective loss of IHCs. Scale bar = 10 μM. (C-F) Schematics of typical cochleograms demonstrating the percent of hair cell loss (IHC and OHC) as a function of the percent distance from the apex of the cochlea at various times after carboplatin was applied to the round window (3, 7, 14 and 28 days later). The basal portion of the cochlea sustained the greatest hair cell loss. [Zhou et al., 2009].

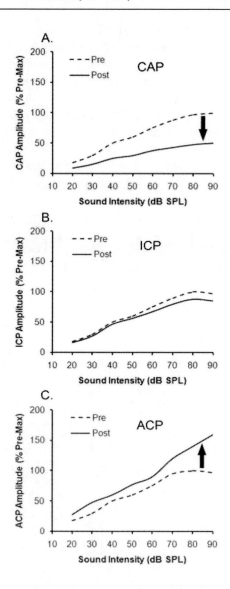

Figure 5. Schematic illustrating typical amplitude-level functions for CAP (A), ICP (B) and ACP (C) recorded before (pre) and ~5 weeks after (post) a moderate dose of carboplatin was administered systemically to chinchillas. Amplitudes are normalized to the maximum pre-treatment response. Following the selective loss of IHCs, there was a significant reduction in the neural input to the central auditory system (i.e., CAP amplitude decreased); however, there was an increase in the ACP amplitude post-treatment, indicative of an increase in central gain. Arrows show the direction of amplitude change at moderate- to high-intensities. [Qiu et al., 2000].

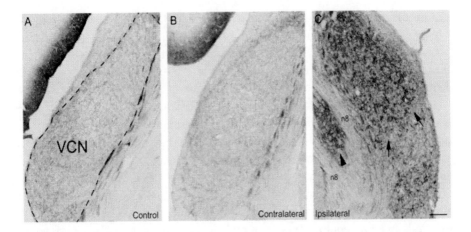

Figure 6. Increased expression of growth associated protein 43 (GAP-43) in the ipsilateral ventral cochlear nucleus (VCN) of the chinchilla 31-days after unilateral application of carboplatin on the round window. Gap-43 was expressed modestly in a control animal (A). In an animal exposed unilaterally to carboplatin, the VCN GAP-43 expression on the untreated side (B) remained at a modest level, whereas the ipsilateral VCN (i.e., exposed side) showed a significant increase in GAP-43 expression (C; darker staining). Staining was darker in the dorsal, high-frequency region than the ventral, low-frequency region (arrows) of the ipsilateral VCN. Also seen in this particular example, is the 8th nerve (n8) surrounding a small area of the VCN (arrowhead), likely due to bifurcation of the fiber bundle. Dashed line in (A) indicates outlines of the VCN. Scale bar = 200 μm. [Kraus et al., 2009].

Studies from several labs, including our own, have provided clues as to the various mechanisms which may underlie the gradual increase in gain in the central auditory system that occurs after carboplatin-induced partial sensory deprivation. Because the enhancement in the ACP amplitude occurred progressively over a period of weeks, this would seem to discount a rapid unmasking of excitatory inputs as a major source of the neuroplasticity. Alternatively, it is possible that the increase in central gain resulted from a gradual change in the release or uptake of excitatory/inhibitory neurotransmitters in the auditory pathway. In support of this possibility, Alkhatib and colleagues [Alkhatib et al., 2006] observed an increase in the number of IC neurons showing monotonic spike rate-level functions, indicative of reduced inhibition, one month after carboplatin-induced peripheral deafferentation. Thus, it is reasonable to suggest that this functional reduction of IC inhibition could manifest as sound-evoked hyperactivity in the AC.

Another possible mechanism contributing to enhanced central gain is an increase in neural convergence via axonal outgrowth and sprouting in the relay nuclei of the auditory pathway. To investigate this possibility, we examined the relationship between the pattern of carboplatin-induced hair cell loss and the location of growth associated protein 43 (GAP-43) immunolabeling in the cochlear nucleus of chinchillas [Kraus et al., 2009]. GAP-43 is a membrane-associated phospho-protein located in axonal growth cones [de Graan et al., 1985], which is highly expressed during neurite outgrowth and early stages of synaptogenesis [Skene and Willard 1981; Mahalik et al., 1992]. Because GAP-43 is largely down-regulated with maturation in most neurons [Skene 1989; Benowitz and Perrone-Bizzozero 1991], its expression can be used effectively as a marker of axonal outgrowth, synaptogenesis and synaptic remodeling [Benowitz and Routtenberg 1997]. Following unilateral application of carboplatin on the round window, IHC loss was distributed throughout the cochlea, whereas OHC degeneration decreased along a base-to-apex gradient. We observed a significant up-regulation of GAP-43 expression in fibers and presynaptic endings in the ipsilateral, but not contralateral, ventral cochlear nucleus (VCN), and no up-regulation in the dorsal cochlear nucleus (DCN) (Figure 6). This up-regulation in the ipsilateral VCN was evident at 15- and 31-days post-carboplatin, but not at earlier time points (3- or 7-days), and it was more pronounced in the dorsal, high-frequency region than the ventral, low-frequency region of the VCN. We suspect that this decreasing gradient of GAP-43 expression from the high- to low-frequency regions in the ipsilateral VCN was the result of the greater hair cell loss in the high-frequency, basal portion of the cochlea. In support of this suggestion, Illing and colleagues [Illing et al., 2005] reported increased GAP-43 expression only in the low-frequency portion of the VCN after restricted surgical ablation of the apical (low-frequency) end of the cochlea in rats.

Why did reactive synaptogenesis occur in the VCN but not DCN? It is unlikely that changes in the auditory nerve were responsible for this disparate expression of GAP-43, as both the VCN and DCN would experience reduced neural input following hair cell loss. Interestingly, a correlation analysis revealed that the loss of OHCs alone or the combination of OHC plus IHC loss was associated with the extent and localization of GAP-43 up-regulation [Kraus et al., 2009]. Thus, it is possible that the source of the fiber sprouting in the VCN arose from specific neurons that lost their postsynaptic targets following the carboplatin-induced OHC damage. Because medial olivocochlear (MOC) neurons project to the cochlea and synapse on OHCs [Warr 1992], and a previous study on rats has shown that MOC neurons contributed to sprouting synapses in VCN expressing GAP-43 after cochlear ablation [Kraus and Illing 2004], we suggest that MOC neurons may be a source of synaptic plasticity in the VCN following unilateral carboplatin exposure in the chinchilla.

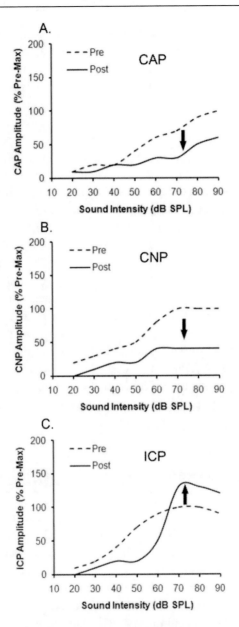

Figure 7. Schematic illustrating typical amplitude-level functions for CAP (A), CNP (B) and ICP (C) at 1 kHz recorded before (pre) and 1-day after (post) acoustic overstimulation (2.8 kHz tone at 105 dB for 2 hours) in the chinchilla. Amplitudes are normalized to the maximum pre-exposure response. Although both the CAP and CNP amplitudes were reduced after the traumatizing tone, there was an increase in the ICP amplitude at moderate- to high-intensities (arrows). [Salvi et al., 1992].

In keeping with this theme, it is relevant to not only discuss the possible functional consequences of the ipsilateral reactive synaptogenesis in the VCN we observed in our recent study [Kraus et al., 2009], but also to address whether synaptic plasticity represents a possible anatomical substrate for the increased central gain we saw after systemic carboplatin treatment [Qiu et al., 2000]. Because the main postsynaptic targets of GAP-43 expression are glutamatergic cells [Illing et al., 1997; Illing et al., 2005], perhaps a strengthening of excitatory neuronal activity in the ipsilateral VCN would help to offset the decrease in sensory input from the damaged ear. By readjusting the signal balance between the two ears, the animal might once again be able to perform binaural processing tasks, such as sound localization in the horizontal plane, which requires signals from both ears to be compared (for review, see [Yin 2002]). Previous studies have shown that horizontal sound localization recovers after hearing loss in laboratory animals [King et al., 2001] and humans [Florentine 1976; Moore 1993]. As to the question of whether or not synaptic plasticity likely contributes to an increase in central gain, it worth noting that, despite differences in our application of carboplatin (round window vs. systemic injection), the time-course of up-regulated expression of GAP-43 [Kraus et al., 2009] was similar to that of the progressive enhancement of the sound-evoked responses in the AC in our original study (i.e., after 2 weeks) [Qiu et al., 2000]. Thus, it seems reasonable to suggest that reactive synaptogenesis in the VCN might contribute to the increase in central gain that occurs after partial sensory deprivation induced by carboplatin ototoxicity.

Acoustic Overstimulation

Of the cochlear insults discussed in this chapter, acoustic overstimulation is the most widely studied. It is well established that acoustic overstimulation preferentially damages the OHCs of the inner ear. Interestingly, we found that chinchillas previously-exposed to a moderate dose of carboplatin, which selectively damaged their IHCs, demonstrated a greater degree of OHC damage following noise exposure than animals that were only exposed to noise [Ding et al., 2004]. This greater susceptibility to OHC damage following the loss of IHCs may have resulted from less olivocochlear efferent feedback and/or a reduction in middle ear muscle attenuation in the inner ear during the noise exposure. A recent review by our colleagues [Henderson et al., 2006] offers a comprehensive description of the various mechanisms underlying noise-induced OHC loss. In this section, we will highlight the electrophysiological changes that we have observed in the auditory pathway following acoustic overstimulation, and how these changes manifest as an increase in central gain. In addition to briefly discussing noise-induced neuroplasticity in the central auditory system, we will present our recent findings on the effect of noise exposure on neurogenesis in the hippocampus.

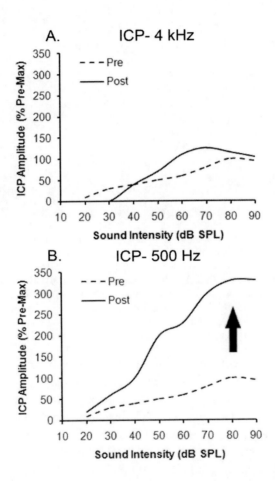

Figure 8. Schematic illustrating typical amplitude-level functions for ICP at 4 kHz (A) and 500 Hz (B) recorded before (pre) and 30-days after (post) acoustic overstimulation (2 kHz tone at 105 dB for 5 days) in the chinchilla. Amplitudes are normalized to the maximum pre-exposure response. Unlike at 4 kHz, the ICP amplitude at 500 Hz was significantly increased at all stimulus intensities (arrow). [Salvi et al., 1990].

DCX

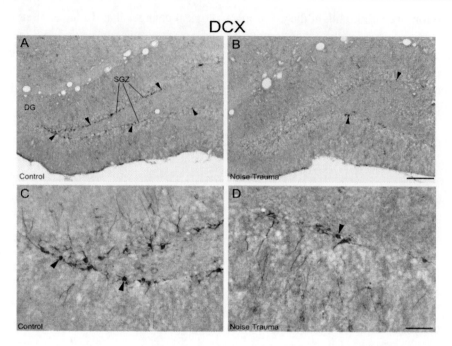

Figure 9. Neuronal precursor cells immunostained for DCX in the adult rat hippocampus in a normal hearing rat (A) and a rat with severe noise trauma 10-weeks after the noise exposure (B). (A) In the normal rat, cell bodies of neuronal precursor cells (arrowheads) form a thin line along the subgranular cell zone (SGZ) in the dentate gyrus (DG). (B) The noise exposed rat showed a strongly reduced number of neuronal precursor cells. Arrowheads point to some of the few remaining cells. (C and D) Single DCX neuronal precursor cells shown at high magnification in the normal hearing rat (C) and in the rat with noise trauma (D). Scale bars: 200 μm in Figure 4B for Figure 4A, B; 50 μm in Figure 4D for Figure 4C, D. [Kraus et al., 2010].

To compare the central versus peripheral effects of noise trauma, we implanted electrodes in the IC, cochlear nucleus (CN) and on the round window, and recorded the sound-evoked local field potentials in the chinchilla before and 1-day after acoustic overstimulation (2.8 kHz tone at 105 dB for 2 hours) [Salvi et al., 1992]. As shown in the schematics of Figure 7, both the CAP and CN potential (CNP) amplitudes were reduced ~50% at high intensities. In contrast, there was an enhancement of the ICP amplitude at sound intensities above 70 dB. These findings are consistent with an increase in central gain following a noise-induced reduction of input from the periphery.

Given that acoustic overstimulation can selectively damage a frequency-specific portion of the cochlea, we were interested in the effect of noise exposure on chinchilla IC responses evoked by sound frequencies both above (4 kHz) and below (500 Hz) that of a traumatizing tone (2 kHz tone at 105 dB for 5 days)

[Salvi et al., 1990]. The acoustic overstimulation resulted in a permanent threshold shift, with the maximum loss at 4 kHz and little to no impairment at low frequencies. As schematized in Figure 8, we found that the ICP amplitudes differed following noise exposure depending on the sound frequency used to evoke the response. For example, 30-days post-exposure, the ICP amplitude at 4 kHz was reduced at low intensities, modestly elevated at intermediate intensities, and relatively unchanged at high intensities. In contrast, the ICP amplitude at 500 Hz was significantly elevated at all intensities, indicative of an increase in IC excitability.

We reasoned that the enhancement of the ICP amplitude at frequencies below that of the acoustic overstimulation may have been caused by a loss of lateral inhibition originating from inputs tuned to high frequencies. To investigate this possibility, we recorded the discharge rates of neurons in the chinchilla IC before and after presenting a traumatizing tone (100-117 dB for 15-30 min) at a frequency above the neurons' characteristic frequencies (CF) [Wang et al., 1996]. Prior to acoustic overstimulation, many IC neurons had sharp tuning curves and non-monotonic spike rate-level functions, both suggestive of strong inhibitory inputs. Following the exposure to the high-frequency tone, there was no change in either the CF threshold or the sharpness of the tuning curve at low intensities of stimulation; however, the tuning curve was broadened at high intensities, the spike rate-level function tended to become more monotonic, and the maximum discharge rate increased. Thus, by damaging the cochlea at frequencies above the neuron's CF, we attenuated the inputs to the neural circuits responsible for lateral inhibition. Taken together, our previous studies identify that frequency-specific lesions to the cochlea can lead to a loss of inhibition in the central auditory system [Wang et al., 1996], which ultimately manifests as an increase in central gain [Salvi et al., 1992] most evident at stimulation frequencies along the low frequency border of the hearing loss [Salvi et al., 1990].

At present, little is known about how intense noise affects brain regions outside of the classical auditory pathway, such as the hippocampus. In addition to playing an important role in learning, memory, mood, and spatial navigation [Squire 1982; Gould et al., 1999; Moscovitch et al., 2005; Becker and Wojtowicz 2007], the hippocampus is a major site of neurogenesis in the adult brain [Altman and Das 1965; Kaplan and Hinds 1977; Kuhn et al., 1996]. For example, in adult rats, ~9000 new cells are born in the hippocampus each day, and most cells differentiate into neurons, form synapses and generate electrical responses [Kaplan and Bell 1984; Cameron et al., 1993; Hastings and Gould 1999; Cameron and McKay 2001; Song et al., 2002; van Praag et al., 2002]. Because the hippocampus responds to auditory stimuli [Bickford-Wimer et al., 1990; Ehlers et al., 1994; Xi et al., 1994; Sakurai 2002], it is susceptible to damage induced by acoustic overstimulation. Previous studies have shown that high-intensity noise can alter the spatial response fields of hippocampal place cells [Goble et al., 2009], and, in the case of very intense blast wave exposure, can even cause the death of granule cells and pyramidal neurons [Saljo et al., 2002].

Recently, we performed the first investigation into the effect of unilateral acoustic overstimulation on neurogenesis in the rat hippocampus [Kraus et al., 2010]. In both noise-exposed rats (narrow-band noise at 126 dB for 2 hours; sacrificed 10 weeks post-exposure) and age-matched controls, we visualized frontal sections of the hippocampus that were immunolabeled for doublecortin (DCX), which identifies neuronal precursor cells, or Ki67, which labels proliferating cells. Figure 9 shows DCX immunopositive neuronal precursor cells and Figure 10 shows Ki67 immunopositive nuclei of proliferating cells in the subgranular zone (SGZ) in the dorsal dentate gyrus. In control rats, we found that DCX-positive cell bodies formed a near continuous band along the SGZ with vertically extending dendrites (Figure 9A, 9C). After noise exposure, however, there was a significant reduction in neuronal precursor cells immunostained for DCX (Figure 9B, 9D), such that the mean DCX cell density was ~72% of that found in the control group. For both control and noise-exposed rats, Ki67 immunolabeled nuclei tended to occur in pairs or small clusters, with only a few Ki67-positive cells present in each frontal section (Figure 10A, 10B). Overall, the mean Ki67 cell density in the noise-exposed rats was reduced to ~57% of the control group mean, indicative of significantly less cell proliferation 10-weeks after the noise exposure. Because memory function may be related to hippocampal neurogenesis [Snyder et al., 2005; Aimone et al., 2006; Winocur et al., 2006; Becker and Wojtowicz 2007], our results suggest that the negative consequences of acoustic overstimulation likely extend beyond impaired auditory processing.

There are a variety of mechanisms that may contribute to the reduced neurogenesis after noise exposure. For example, similar to granule cells and pyramidal neurons [Saljo et al., 2002], the number of DCX-positive cells could be reduced by noise-induced cell death. Given that we observed a decrease in Ki67 cell density, it is possible that the reduced DCX population resulted from a decreased rate of cell proliferation. Following noise-exposure, neurogenesis may have been impaired due to the increased stress associated with hearing loss. Finally, it is possible that, similar to the central auditory system, noise-induced cochlear damage caused long-term hyperactivity in the hippocampus, which in turn resulted in the suppressed neurogenesis we observed 10-weeks post-exposure.

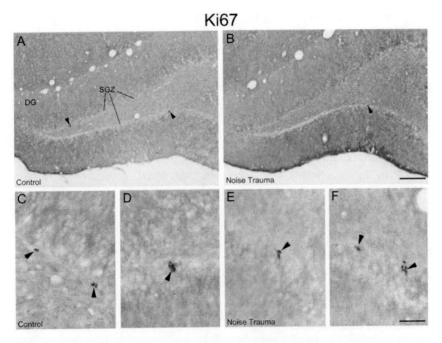

Figure 10. Dividing cells immunostained for Ki67 in the adult rat hippocampus in a normal hearing rat (A, C and D) and a rat with severe noise trauma 10-weeks after the noise exposure (B, E and F). (A and B) In the normal rat as well as the noise-exposed rat, Ki67-immunopositive nuclei (arrowheads) are present in the subgranular cell zone (SGZ) in the dentate gyrus (DG). Ki67 immunopositive cells were typically clustered in pairs or small groups in normal hearing rats (C and D) as well as in noise exposed rats (E and F). Scale bars: 200 µm in Figure 5B for Figure 5A, B; 50 µm in Figure 5F for Figure 5C–F. [Kraus et al., 2010].

Conclusion

Hearing loss resulting from noise exposure and ototoxic drugs has been traditionally thought to be a cochlear phenomenon associated with the death of hair cells, supporting cells and spiral ganglion neurons. The net result of the various forms of cochlear damage is a reduced neural input to the central nervous system. Our results indicate that the central nervous system does not respond passively to the lack of input, but rather turns up its gain in order to compensate for a reduced neural input. It is not entirely clear where exactly along the central auditory pathway the mechanisms underlying auditory signal gain reside; our data suggest gain increases are likely to occur in the auditory brainstem as well as midbrain and cortical levels. Further research is needed to identify the full range of mechanisms that enhance the gain of the central auditory pathway. The central gain changes described in this chapter most likely play a critical role in the normal optimization of auditory perception as a result of dynamic changes that occur during development (e.g., change in head size) and aging (i.e., central degeneration and atrophy); however, these mechanisms may become hypervigilent following extensive peripheral hearing loss resulting in pathological consequences for auditory processing. Finally, our recent observations showing that noise-induced hearing loss suppresses neurogenesis in the hippocampus serves to reinforce the notion that the ear and auditory system are linked to complicated, interconnected brain networks involved in the recognition and interpretation of sounds. What we hear and perceive is not only dependent on the classical auditory pathway, but also extensive neural networks widely distributed throughout the central nervous system including other sensory, motor, and cognitive systems.

Acknowledgments

Supported in part by grants from Tinnitus Research Initiative (TRI), Royal National Institute for Deaf People (RNID), and National Institutes of Health (NIH; R01DC00909101, R01DC009219-01).

References

Aimone, J. B., Wiles, J. & Gage, F. H. (2006). Potential role for adult neurogenesis in the encoding of time in new memories. *Nat Neurosci 9*: 723-727.

Alkhatib, A., Biebel, U. W. & Smolders, J. W. (2006). Reduction of inhibition in the inferior colliculus after inner hair cell loss. *Neuroreport 17*: 1493-1497.

Altman, J. & Das, G. D. (1965). Autoradiographic and histological evidence of postnatal hippocampal neurogenesis in rats. *J Comp Neurol 124*: 319-335.

Becker, S. & Wojtowicz, J. M. (2007). A model of hippocampal neurogenesis in memory and mood disorders. *Trends Cogn Sci 11*: 70-76.

Benowitz, L. I. & Perrone-Bizzozero, N. I. (1991). The expression of GAP-43 in relation to neuronal growth and plasticity: when, where, how, and why? *Prog Brain Res 89*: 69-87.

Benowitz, L. I. & Routtenberg, A. (1997). GAP-43: an intrinsic determinant of neuronal development and plasticity. *Trends Neurosci 20*: 84-91.

Bickford-Wimer, P. C., Nagamoto, H., Johnson, R., Adler, L. E., Egan, M., Rose, G. M. & Freedman, R. (1990). Auditory sensory gating in hippocampal neurons: a model system in the rat. *Biol Psychiatry 27*: 183-192.

Bortner, C. D. & Cidlowski, J. A. (1998). A necessary role for cell shrinkage in apoptosis. *Biochem Pharmacol 56*: 1549-1559.

Brownell, W. E. (1990). Outer hair cell electromotility and otoacoustic emissions. *Ear Hear 11*: 82-92.

Cameron, H. A. & McKay, R. D. (2001). Adult neurogenesis produces a large pool of new granule cells in the dentate gyrus. *J Comp Neurol 435*: 406-417.

Cameron, H. A., Woolley, C. S., McEwen, B. S. & Gould, E. (1993). Differentiation of newly born neurons and glia in the dentate gyrus of the adult rat. *Neuroscience 56*: 337-344.

Cazals, Y. (2000). Auditory sensori-neural alterations induced by salicylate. *Prog Neurobiol 62*: 583-631.

Chen, G. D., Kermany, M. H., D'Elia, A., Ralli, M., Tanaka, C., Bielefeld, E. C., Ding, D., Henderson, D. & Salvi, R. (2010). Too much of a good thing: long-term treatment with salicylate strengthens outer hair cell function but impairs auditory neural activity. *Hear Res 265*: 63-69.

Dallos, P. & Harris, D. (1978). Properties of auditory nerve responses in absence of outer hair cells. *J Neurophysiol 41*: 365-383.

de Graan, P. N., van Hooff, C. O., Tilly, B. C., Oestreicher, A. B., Schotman, P. & Gispen, W. H. (1985). Phosphoprotein B-50 in nerve growth cones from fetal rat brain. *Neurosci Lett 61*: 235-241.

Ding, D., Jiang, H., Wang, J., Yang, J., McFadden, S. L. & Salvi, R. J. (2004). Inner hair cell missing potentiates noise induced outer hair cell lesion. *Journal of Audiology and Speech Pathology 12*: 413-415.

Ding, D. L., Wang, J., Salvi, R., Henderson, D., Hu, B. H., McFadden, S. L. & Mueller, M. (1999). Selective loss of inner hair cells and type-I ganglion neurons in carboplatin-treated chinchillas. Mechanisms of damage and protection. *Ann N Y Acad Sci 884*: 152-170.

Eggermont, J. J. & Roberts, L. E. (2004). The neuroscience of tinnitus. *Trends Neurosci 27*: 676-682.

Ehlers, C. L., Kaneko, W. M., Robledo, P. & Lopez, A. L. (1994). Long-latency event-related potentials in rats: effects of task and stimulus parameters. *Neuroscience 62*: 759-769.

Ermilov, S. A., Murdock, D. R., El-Daye, D., Brownell, W. E. & Anvari, B. (2005). Effects of salicylate on plasma membrane mechanics. *J Neurophysiol 94*: 2105-2110.

Florentine, M. (1976). Relation between lateralization and loudness in asymmetrical hearing losses. *J Am Audiol Soc 1*: 243-251.

Friis, M. B., Friborg, C. R., Schneider, L., Nielsen, M. B., Lambert, I. H., Christensen, S. T. & Hoffmann, E. K. (2005). Cell shrinkage as a signal to apoptosis in NIH 3T3 fibroblasts. *J Physiol 567*: 427-443.

Gao, W. Q. (1999). Role of neurotrophins and lectins in prevention of ototoxicity. *Ann N Y Acad Sci 884*: 312-327.

Gerken, G. M. (1996). Central tinnitus and lateral inhibition: an auditory brainstem model. *Hear Res 97*: 75-83.

Goble, T. J., Moller, A. R. & Thompson, L. T. (2009). Acute high-intensity sound exposure alters responses of place cells in hippocampus. *Hear Res 253*: 52-59.

Gould, E., Tanapat, P., Hastings, N. B. & Shors, T. J. (1999). Neurogenesis in adulthood: a possible role in learning. *Trends Cogn Sci 3*: 186-192.

Hastings, N. B. & Gould, E. (1999). Rapid extension of axons into the CA3 region by adult-generated granule cells. *J Comp Neurol 413*: 146-154.

Henderson, D., Bielefeld, E. C., Harris, K. C. & Hu, B. H. (2006). The role of oxidative stress in noise-induced hearing loss. *Ear Hear 27*: 1-19.

Hofstetter, P., Ding, D. & Salvi, R. (1997). Magnitude and pattern of inner and outer hair cell loss in chinchilla as a function of carboplatin dose. *Audiology 36*: 301-311.

Huang, Z. W., Luo, Y., Wu, Z., Tao, Z., Jones, R. O. & Zhao, H. B. (2005). Paradoxical enhancement of active cochlear mechanics in long-term administration of salicylate. *J Neurophysiol 93*: 2053-2061.

Illing, R. B., Horvath, M. & Laszig, R. (1997). Plasticity of the auditory brainstem: effects of cochlear ablation on GAP-43 immunoreactivity in the rat. *J Comp Neurol 382*: 116-138.

Illing, R. B., Kraus, K. S. & Meidinger, M. A. (2005). Reconnecting neuronal networks in the auditory brainstem following unilateral deafening. *Hear Res 206*: 185-199.

Ison, J. R., Allen, P. D. & O'Neill, W. E. (2007). Age-related hearing loss in C57BL/6J mice has both frequency-specific and non-frequency-specific components that produce a hyperacusis-like exaggeration of the acoustic startle reflex. *J Assoc Res Otolaryngol 8*: 539-550.

Kaplan, M. S. & Bell, D. H. (1984). Mitotic neuroblasts in the 9-day-old and 11-month-old rodent hippocampus. *J Neurosci 4*: 1429-1441.

Kaplan, M. S. & Hinds, J. W. (1977). Neurogenesis in the adult rat: electron microscopic analysis of light radioautographs. *Science 197*: 1092-1094.

King, A. J., Kacelnik, O., Mrsic-Flogel, T. D., Schnupp, J. W., Parsons, C. H. & Moore, D. R. (2001). How plastic is spatial hearing? *Audiol Neurootol 6*: 182-186.

Kraus, K. S., Ding, D., Zhou, Y. & Salvi, R. J. (2009). Central auditory plasticity after carboplatin-induced unilateral inner ear damage in the chinchilla: up-regulation of GAP-43 in the ventral cochlear nucleus. *Hear Res 255*: 33-43.

Kraus, K. S. & Illing, R. B. (2004). Superior olivary contributions to auditory system plasticity: medial but not lateral olivocochlear neurons are the source of cochleotomy-induced GAP-43 expression in the ventral cochlear nucleus. *J Comp Neurol 475*: 374-390.

Kraus, K. S., Mitra, S., Jimenez, Z., Hinduja, S., Ding, D., Jiang, H., Gray, L., Lobarinas, E., Sun, W. & Salvi, R. J. (2010). Noise trauma impairs neurogenesis in the rat hippocampus. *Neuroscience 167*: 1216-1226.

Kuhn, H. G., Dickinson-Anson, H. & Gage, F. H. (1996). Neurogenesis in the dentate gyrus of the adult rat: age-related decrease of neuronal progenitor proliferation. *J Neurosci 16*: 2027-2033.

Maeno, E., Ishizaki, Y., Kanaseki, T., Hazama, A. & Okada, Y. (2000). Normotonic cell shrinkage because of disordered volume regulation is an early prerequisite to apoptosis. *Proc Natl Acad Sci U S A 97*: 9487-9492.

Mahalik, T. J., Carrier, A., Owens, G. P. & Clayton, G. (1992). The expression of GAP43 mRNA during the late embryonic and early postnatal development of the CNS of the rat: an in situ hybridization study. *Brain Res Dev Brain Res 67*: 75-83.

Moore, D. R. (1993). Plasticity of binaural hearing and some possible mechanisms following late-onset deprivation. *J Am Acad Audiol 4*: 277-283; discussion 283-274.

Moscovitch, M., Rosenbaum, R. S., Gilboa, A., Addis, D. R., Westmacott, R., Grady, C., McAndrews, M. P., Levine, B., Black, S., Winocur, G. & Nadel, L. (2005). Functional neuroanatomy of remote episodic, semantic and spatial memory: a unified account based on multiple trace theory. *J Anat 207*: 35-66.

Muller, M., Klinke, R., Arnold, W. & Oestreicher, E. (2003). Auditory nerve fibre responses to salicylate revisited. *Hear Res 183*: 37-43.

Neumahr, S., Hapfelmeier, G., Scheller, M., Schneck, H., Franke, C. & Kochs, E. (2000). Dual action of isoflurane on the gamma-aminobutyric acid (GABA)-mediated currents through recombinant alpha(1)beta(2)gamma(2L)-GABA(A)-receptor channels. *Anesth Analg 90*: 1184-1190.

Okada, Y., Maeno, E., Shimizu, T., Dezaki, K., Wang, J. & Morishima, S. (2001). Receptor-mediated control of regulatory volume decrease (RVD) and apoptotic volume decrease (AVD). *J Physiol 532*: 3-16.

Qiu, C., Salvi, R., Ding, D. & Burkard, R. (2000). Inner hair cell loss leads to enhanced response amplitudes in auditory cortex of unanesthetized chinchillas: evidence for increased system gain. *Hear Res 139*: 153-171.

Ralli, M., Lobarinas, E., Fetoni, A. R., Stolzberg, D., Paludetti, G. & Salvi, R. (2010). Comparison of Salicylate- and Quinine-Induced Tinnitus in Rats: Development, Time Course, and Evaluation of Audiologic Correlates. *Otol Neurotol.*

Ranft, A., Kurz, J., Deuringer, M., Haseneder, R., Dodt, H. U., Zieglgansberger, W., Kochs, E., Eder, M. & Hapfelmeier, G. (2004). Isoflurane modulates glutamatergic and GABAergic neurotransmission in the amygdala. *Eur J Neurosci 20*: 1276-1280.

Ruel, J., Chabbert, C., Nouvian, R., Bendris, R., Eybalin, M., Leger, C. L., Bourien, J., Mersel, M. & Puel, J. L. (2008). Salicylate enables cochlear arachidonic-acid-sensitive NMDA receptor responses. *J Neurosci 28*: 7313-7323.

Ryan, A. & Dallos, P. (1975). Effect of absence of cochlear outer hair cells on behavioural auditory threshold. *Nature 253*: 44-46.

Ryan, A., Dallos, P. & McGee, T. (1979). Psychophysical tuning curves and auditory thresholds after hair cell damage in the chinchilla. *J Acoust Soc Am 66*: 370-378.

Saito, T., Saito, H., Saito, K., Wakui, S., Manabe, Y. & Tsuda, G. (1989). Ototoxicity of carboplatin in guinea pigs. *Auris Nasus Larynx 16*: 13-21.

Sakurai, Y. (2002). Coding of auditory temporal and pitch information by hippocampal individual cells and cell assemblies in the rat. *Neuroscience 115*: 1153-1163.

Saljo, A., Bao, F., Jingshan, S., Hamberger, A., Hansson, H. A. & Haglid, K. G. (2002). Exposure to short-lasting impulse noise causes neuronal c-Jun expression and induction of apoptosis in the adult rat brain. *J Neurotrauma 19*: 985-991.

Salvi, R. J., Powers, N. L., Saunders, S. S., Boettcher, F. A. & Clock, A. E. (1992). Enhancement of evoked response amplitude and single unit activity after noise exposure. A. Dancer, D. Henderson, R. J. Salvi & R. Hamernik. *Noise-Induced Hearing Loss.* (156-171). St. Louis, MO: Mosby Year Book.

Salvi, R. J., Saunders, S. S., Gratton, M. A., Arehole, S. & Powers, N. (1990). Enhanced evoked response amplitudes in the inferior colliculus of the chinchilla following acoustic trauma. *Hear Res 50*: 245-257.

Salvi, R. J., Wang, J. & Ding, D. (2000). Auditory plasticity and hyperactivity following cochlear damage. *Hear Res 147*: 261-274.

Schmiedt, R. A., Zwislocki, J. J. & Hamernik, R. P. (1980). Effects of hair cell lesions on responses of cochlear nerve fibers. I. Lesions, tuning curves, two-tone inhibition, and responses to trapezoidal-wave patterns. *J Neurophysiol* 43: 1367-1389.

Schuknecht, H. F. (1994). Auditory and cytocochlear correlates of inner ear disorders. *Otolaryngol Head Neck Surg 110*: 530-538.

Skene, J. H. (1989). Axonal growth-associated proteins. *Annu Rev Neurosci 12*: 127-156.

Skene, J. H. & Willard, M. (1981). Changes in axonally transported proteins during axon regeneration in toad retinal ganglion cells. *J Cell Biol 89*: 86-95.

Snyder, J. S., Hong, N. S., McDonald, R. J. & Wojtowicz, J. M. (2005). A role for adult neurogenesis in spatial long-term memory. *Neuroscience 130*: 843-852.

Song, H. J., Stevens, C. F. & Gage, F. H. (2002). Neural stem cells from adult hippocampus develop essential properties of functional CNS neurons. *Nat Neurosci 5*: 438-445.

Squire, L. R. (1982). The neuropsychology of human memory. *Annu Rev Neurosci 5*: 241-273.

Starr, A., Picton, T. W., Sininger, Y., Hood, L. J. & Berlin, C. I. (1996). Auditory neuropathy. *Brain 119 (Pt 3)*: 741-753.

Sun, W., Lu, J., Stolzberg, D., Gray, L., Deng, A., Lobarinas, E. & Salvi, R. J. (2009). Salicylate increases the gain of the central auditory system. *Neuroscience 159*: 325-334.

Trautwein, P., Hofstetter, P., Wang, J., Salvi, R. & Nostrant, A. (1996). Selective inner hair cell loss does not alter distortion product otoacoustic emissions. *Hear Res 96*: 71-82.

Tunstall, M. J., Gale, J. E. & Ashmore, J. F. (1995). Action of salicylate on membrane capacitance of outer hair cells from the guinea-pig cochlea. *J Physiol 485 (Pt 3)*: 739-752.

Turner, J. G. & Parrish, J. (2008). Gap detection methods for assessing salicylate-induced tinnitus and hyperacusis in rats. *Am J Audiol 17*: S185-192.

van Praag, H., Schinder, A. F., Christie, B. R., Toni, N., Palmer, T. D. & Gage, F. H. (2002). Functional neurogenesis in the adult hippocampus. *Nature 415*: 1030-1034.

Wake, M., Takeno, S., Ibrahim, D. & Harrison, R. (1994). Selective inner hair cell ototoxicity induced by carboplatin. *Laryngoscope 104*: 488-493.

Wang, H. T., Luo, B., Huang, Y. N., Zhou, K. Q. & Chen, L. (2008). Sodium salicylate suppresses serotonin-induced enhancement of GABAergic spontaneous inhibitory postsynaptic currents in rat inferior colliculus in vitro. *Hear Res 236*: 42-51.

Wang, H. T., Luo, B., Zhou, K. Q., Xu, T. L. & Chen, L. (2006). Sodium salicylate reduces inhibitory postsynaptic currents in neurons of rat auditory cortex. *Hear Res 215*: 77-83.

Wang, J., Powers, N. L., Hofstetter, P., Trautwein, P., Ding, D. & Salvi, R. (1997). Effects of selective inner hair cell loss on auditory nerve fiber threshold, tuning and spontaneous and driven discharge rate. *Hear Res 107*: 67-82.

Wang, J., Salvi, R. J. & Powers, N. (1996). Plasticity of response properties of inferior colliculus neurons following acute cochlear damage. *J Neurophysiol 75*: 171-183.

Warr, W. B. (1992). Organization of olivocochlear efferent systems in mammals. D. B. Webster, N. N. Popper & R. R. Fay. *The Mammalian Auditory Pathway: Neuroanatomy.* (410-448). New York: Springer Verlag.

Wei, L., Ding, D. & Salvi, R. (2010). Salicylate-induced degeneration of cochlea spiral ganglion neurons-apoptosis signaling. *Neuroscience 168*: 288-299.

Winocur, G., Wojtowicz, J. M., Sekeres, M., Snyder, J. S. & Wang, S. (2006). Inhibition of neurogenesis interferes with hippocampus-dependent memory function. *Hippocampus 16*: 296-304.

Wyllie, A. H., Kerr, J. F. & Currie, A. R. (1980). Cell death: the significance of apoptosis. *Int Rev Cytol 68*: 251-306.

Xi, M. C., Woody, C. D. & Gruen, E. (1994). Identification of short latency auditory responsive neurons in the cat dentate nucleus. *Neuroreport 5*: 1567-1570.

Yang, G., Lobarinas, E., Zhang, L., Turner, J., Stolzberg, D., Salvi, R. & Sun, W. (2007). Salicylate induced tinnitus: behavioral measures and neural activity in auditory cortex of awake rats. *Hear Res 226*: 244-253.

Yang, K., Huang, Z. W., Liu, Z. Q., Xiao, B. K. & Peng, J. H. (2009). Long-term administration of salicylate enhances prestin expression in rat cochlea. *Int J Audiol 48*: 18-23.

Yin, T. C. T. (2002). Neuronal mechanics of encoding binaural sound localization cues in the auditory brainstem. D. Oertel, R. R. Fay & A. N. Popper. *Integrative Functions in the Mammalian Auditory Pathway.* (99-159). New York: Springer Verlag.

Zhi, M., Ratnanather, J. T., Ceyhan, E., Popel, A. S. & Brownell, W. E. (2007). Hypotonic swelling of salicylate-treated cochlear outer hair cells. *Hear Res 228*: 95-104.

Zhou, Y., Ding, D., Kraus, K. S., Yu, D. & Salvi, R. J. (2009). Functional and structural changes in the chinchilla cochlea and vestibular system following round window application of carboplatin. *Audiol Med 7*: 189-199.

Index

D

T